AF652950

Sports Nutrition

Vijaya Lakshmi

KHEL SAHITYA KENDRA
7/26, Ansari Road, Daryaganj,
New Delhi-110002

Published by:
KHEL SAHITYA KENDRA
7/26, Ansari Road, Darya Ganj, New Delhi-110002
Ph.: (O) 011-43551324, 42564726, 47090343
(M) 9811088729, (Fax) 011-42564726
(Res.) 47091605
E-mail: khelsahitya1@rediffmail.com
Website: www.khelsahitya.com, www.kskpublisher.com

© 2026 - All Rights Reserved

ISBN 978-81-7524-175-6

PRINTED IN INDIA 2026

No part of this publication may be re-produced, stored in a retrieval system or published/distributed in any form or by any means, electronic, mechanical, photocopying, recording, scanning, web or otherwise without the written permission of the Publisher. Publisher has obtained all the information in this book from the sources believed to be reliable and true. However, Publisher or its editors or illustrators don't take any reponsibility for the absolute accuracy of any information published, and the damages or loss suffered thereupon.

All disputes subject to Delhi jurisdiction only.

Printed by:
ASIAN OFFSET PRINTERS
Delhi

Laser Typesetting by:
K.S.K. DTP UNIT, DELHI

I DEDICATE THIS BOOK TO MY FATHER LATE SH. T. N. RAMA KRISHNAN WHO ALWAYS MOTIVATED ME SINCE MY CHILDHOOD TO ACHIEVE SOMETHING GOOD WITHIN IN MY LIFE TIME. HIS BLESSINGS ARE ALWAYS WITH ME AND I AM SURE TO SUCCEED IN EACH AND EVERY ASSIGNMENT I INVOLVE.

VIJAYA LAKSHMI

Sports Nutrition

CHAPTER 1

OVERVIEW OF NUTRITION

Nutrition is the process of consuming, absorbing, and using nutrients needed by the body for growth, development, and the maintenance of life; nutrients are chemical substances in foods that nourish the body.

Many nutrients can be synthesized in the body. Those that cannot be synthesized in the body called essential nutrients-must be consumed in the diet. They include amino acids (in proteins), certain fatty acids (in fats and oils), minerals, and vitamins. Nine of the 20 amino acids in proteins are essential nutrients.If essential nutrients are not supplied in the quantities required, nutritional deficiency disorders may result. To determine whether a person is getting enough nutrients, a doctor asks about eating habits and diet, performs a physical examination to assess the composition (the amount of fat and muscle) and functioning of the body, and orders laboratory tests to measure the nutrient content of blood and tissues.

Generally, nutrients are divided into two classes: macronutrients and micronutrients. Macronutrients, which include proteins, fats, carbohydrates, and some minerals, are required daily in large quantities. They constitute the bulk of the diet and supply the energy and building blocks needed for growth, maintenance, and activity. Micronutrients are required in small quantities milligrams (one thousandth of a gram) to micrograms (one millionth of a gram). They include vitamins and trace minerals that catalyze the utilization of macronutrients. Other useful components of food aren't digested or metabolized to any appreciable extent. These components include some fibers, such as cellulose, pectin, and gums. Authorities recommend that 20 grams of fiber be consumed daily to improve movement in the gastrointestinal tract, moderate the changes in blood sugar and cholesterol that occur after meals, and increase the elimination of cancer-causing substances produced by the bacteria in the large intestine. Food additives such as preservatives, emulsifiers, anti-oxidants, and stabilizers improve the production, processing, storage, and packaging of foods. Substances such as spices, flavors, odors, colors, phytochemicals (nonnutrients in plants, which have biologic activity in animals), and many other natural products improve the appearance, taste, and stability of food. Food in the daily diet contains as many as 100,000 substances, of which only 300 are nutrients and 45 are essential nutrients.

Macronutrients

The organic macronutrients are carbohydrates, fats, and proteins, which supply 90 percent of the dry weight of the diet and 100 percent of its energy. They are digested in the intestine and broken down into their basic units: sugars from carbohydrates, fatty acids and glycerol from fats, and amino acids from proteins. The energy content is 4 calories in a gram of protein or carbohydrate and 9 calories in a gram of fat (1 gram equals 1/28 of an ounce). As sources of energy, carbohydrates, fats, and proteins are interchangeable in proportion to their energy content.

Energy intake varies markedly from about 1,000 to more than 4,000 calories a day depending on age, sex, and physical activity. Typically, sedentary women, young children, and older adults need about 1,600 calories a day; older children, active adult women, and sedentary men need about 2,000 calories; and active adolescent boys and young men need about 2,400 calories. About 55 percent of the calories commonly come from carbohydrates, about 30 percent from fats, and about 15 percent from proteins. If the energy intake is insufficient for the body's needs, weight loss occurs, and fat stored in the body and to a lesser degree protein is used to supply the energy needed. Total starvation causes death in 8 to 12 weeks.

The essential fatty acids make up about 7 percent of the fat consumed in a normal diet (which is 3 percent of the total calories or about 8 grams) and thus are considered macronutrients. They include linoleic acid, linolenic acid, arachidonic acid, eicosapentaenoic acid, and docosahexaenoic acid. Linoleic acid and linolenic acid are found in vegetable oils; eicosapentaenoic acid and docosahexaenoic acid, which are essential for brain development, are found in fish oils. In the body, arachidonic acid can be formed from linoleic acid, and eicosapentaenoic and docosahexaenoic acid can be formed from linolenic acid, although fish oil is a more efficient source.

The macrominerals are calcium, phosphorus, sodium, chloride, potassium, and magnesium. They are considered macronutrients because they are required in fairly large quantities (about 1 or 2 grams a day). Water, also a macronutrient, is required in amounts of 1 milliliter for each calorie of energy expended or about 2,500 milliliters (2.6 quarts) a day.

Micronutrients

Vitamins and trace minerals are micronutrients. Vitamins are classified as water soluble (vitamin C and eight members of the vitamin B complex) or fat soluble (vitamins A, D, E, and K).

Essential trace minerals include iron, zinc, copper, manganese, molybdenum, selenium, iodide, and fluoride. Except for fluoride, all of these minerals activate enzymes required in metabolism. Fluoride forms a stable compound with calcium, helping stabilize the mineral content of bones and teeth and helping prevent tooth decay. Trace minerals such as arsenic, chromium, cobalt, nickel, silicon, and vanadium, which may be essential in animal nutrition, have not been established as requirements in human nutrition. All trace minerals are toxic at high levels, and some (arsenic, nickel, and chromium) have been identified as causes of cancer.

Nutritional Requirements

The objective of a proper diet is to achieve and maintain a desirable body composition and a large capacity for physical and mental work. The daily requirements for essential nutrients depend on a person's age, sex, height, weight, and metabolic and physical activity.

The U.S. Department of Agriculture originally proposed the basic four food groups (dairy products, meat and protein-rich vegetables, cereals and breads, and fruits and vegetables) as a guide to a balanced diet, but currently it suggests that the food guide pyramid is a better guide. This guide is intended to help people choose a diet that supplies essential nutrients as well as helps reduce the risk of such disorders as cancer, high blood pressure, coronary artery disease, and strokes. In this guide, the number of servings a day for each food group varies, depending on energy needs that range from 1,600 to more than 2,400 calories a day. For example, a person who consumes 1,600 calories a day could eat 6 servings from the bread group and 3 from the vegetable group, whereas a person who consumes 2,400 calories a day could eat 10 servings from the bread group and 5 from the vegetable group. In general, the consumption of fat should be reduced to about 30 percent of calories, and the consumption of fruits, vegetables, and cereals should be increased.

Malnutrition

Malnutrition can result from either undernutrition or overnutrition. Both conditions are caused by an imbalance between the body's need for and the intake of essential nutrients.

Undernutrition, a deficiency of essential nutrients, can result from inadequate intake because of a poor diet or poor absorption from the intestine (malabsorption); abnormally high usage of nutrients by the body; or abnormal loss of nutrients through diarrhea, bleeding (hemorrhage), kidney failure, or excessive sweating. Overnutrition, an excess of essential nutrients, can result from overeating, excessive use of vitamins or other supplements, or underexercising.

Malnutrition develops in stages: First, changes occur in the levels of nutrients in blood and tissues, then changes occur in enzyme levels, next body organs and tissues malfunction, and then symptoms of illness and death occur.

The body needs more nutrients during certain stages of life, particularly in infancy, early childhood, and adolescence; during pregnancy; and while breastfeeding. In old age, nutritional needs are lower, but the ability to absorb nutrients is often reduced. Therefore, the risk of undernutrition is greater at these times of life, and even more so among people who are economically deprived.

Nutritional Assessment

Height & Weight Reference Chart for Adults

Height Weight (Pounds)

	Women	Men
4' 10"	92-121	--
4' 11"	95-124	--
5' 0"	98-127	--
5' 1"	101-130	105-134
5' 2"	104-134	108-137
5' 3"	107-138	111-141
5' 4"	110-142	114-145
5' 5"	114-146	117-149
5' 6"	118-150	121-154
5' 7"	122-154	125-159
5' 8"	126-159	129-163
5' 9"	130-164	133-167
5' 10"	134-169	137-172
5' 11"	--	141-177
6' 0"	--	145-182
6' 1"	--	149-187
6' 2"	--	153-192
6' 3"	--	157-197

*Height is without shoes; weight is without clothes.

To assess a person's nutritional status, a doctor asks about diet and medical problems, performs a physical examination, and orders certain laboratory tests. Blood levels of nutrients and substances that depend on nutrient levels (such as hemoglobin, thyroid hormones, and transferrin) are measured.

To determine a person's diet history, the doctor asks what foods were eaten in the previous 24 hours and what types of food are usually eaten. The person may be asked to keep a food diary, in which he lists everything he eats for 3 days. During the physical examination, the doctor observes the person's general appearance and behavior as well as the distribution of body fat and assesses the functioning of body organs.

Nutritional deficiencies can cause a number of medical problems. For example, gastrointestinal bleeding can cause iron deficiency anemia. A person being treated with high doses of vitamin A for acne may develop headaches and double vision as a result of vitamin A toxicity. Any body system can be affected by a nutritional disorder. For example, the nervous system is affected by niacin deficiency (pellagra), beriberi, vitamin B6 (pyridoxine) deficiency or excess, and vitamin B12 deficiency. Taste and smell are affected by zinc deficiency. The cardiovascular system is affected by beriberi, obesity, a high-fat diet leading to hypercholesterolemia and coronary artery disease, and a high-salt diet leading to hypertension. The gastrointestinal tract is affected by pellagra, folic acid deficiency, and alcoholism. The mouth (lips, tongue, gums, and mucous membranes) is affected by a deficiency of B vitamins and scurvy. An enlarged thyroid gland may result from iodine deficiency. A tendency to bleed and skin symptoms such as rashes, dryness, and swelling from fluid retention (edema) can occur in scurvy, vitamin K deficiency, vitamin A deficiency, and beriberi. Bones and joints are affected by rickets, osteomalacia, osteoporosis, and scurvy.

A person's nutritional status can be determined in several ways. One is to measure height and weight and compare them with those in standardized tables. Another way is to calculate body mass index—the weight (in kilograms) divided by height (in meters squared). A body mass index of 20 to 25 is generally considered normal for men and women.

Still another way to assess nutritional status is by measuring skinfold thickness. A fold of skin on the back of the upper arm (the triceps skinfold) is pulled away from the arm so the layer of fat beneath the skin can be measured, usually with a caliper. Fat beneath the skin accounts for 50 percent of body fat. A skinfold measurement of about ½ inch in men and about 1 inch in women is considered normal.

Nutritional status can also be assessed by measuring the circumference of the left upper arm to estimate the amount of skeletal muscle in the body (lean body mass).

X-rays can help determine bone density and the condition of the heart and lungs. They can also detect gastrointestinal disturbances caused by malnutrition.

When a doctor suspects severe malnutrition, he may order a complete blood cell count and blood and urine tests to measure levels of vitamins, minerals, and waste products such as urea. Skin tests may also be ordered to assess certain types of immunity.

Risk Factors

Infants and children are at particular risk for undernutrition because they need a greater amount of calories and nutrients for growth and development. They may develop deficiencies in iron, folic acid, vitamin C, and copper from inadequate diets. Insufficient intake of protein, calories, and other nutrients can lead to protein-energy malnutrition, a particularly severe form of undernutrition that retards growth and development. A bleeding tendency in newborns (hemorrhagic disease of the newborn) caused by a deficiency of vitamin K can be life threatening. As children approach adolescence, their nutritional requirements increase because their growth rate increases.

A woman who is pregnant or breastfeeding has an increased need for all nutrients to prevent malnutrition in herself and her baby. Folic acid supplements are recommended during pregnancy to reduce the risk of brain or spinal defects (spina bifida) in the baby. Although women who have taken oral contraceptives are more likely to develop folic acid deficiency, there is no proof that the fetus will be deficient. The baby of an alcoholic woman may be physically and mentally impaired by fetal alcohol syndrome, because alcohol abuse and the resulting malnutrition affect fetal development. An infant who is breastfed exclusively can develop vitamin B12 deficiency if the mother is a vegetarian who eats no animal products (a vegan).

Elderly people may become malnourished because of loneliness, physical and mental handicaps, immobility, or chronic illness. In addition, their ability to absorb nutrients is reduced, possibly contributing to such problems as iron deficiency anemia, osteoporosis, and osteomalacia.

Aging is accompanied by a progressive loss of muscle that's unrelated to any disease or dietary deficiency. This loss averages about 22 pounds for men and 11 pounds for women. It accounts for the slowdown that occurs in metabolism, the decrease in total body weight, and the increase in body fat from about 20 to 30 percent in men and 27 to 40 percent in women. Because of tnese changes and a reduction in physical activity, older people need fewer calories and less protein than younger people do.

Who Is at Risk for Overnutrition?

- Children and adults who have good appetites but don't exercise
- People who are more than 20 percent overweight
- People on high-fat, high-salt diets
- People who take high doses of nicotinic acid (niacin). for hypercholesterolemia
- Women who take high doses of vitamin B6 (pyridoxine) for premenstrual syndrome
- People who take high doses of vitamin A for skin disorders
- People who take high doses of iron or other trace minerals without a prescription

People who have a chronic disease that causes malabsorption tend to have trouble absorbing fat-soluble vitamins (A, D, E, and K), vitamin B12, calcium, and iron. Liver disease impairs the storage of vitamins A and B12 and interferes with the metabolism of protein and glucose, a type of sugar. People who have kidney disease, including those on dialysis, are prone to deficiencies of protein, iron, and vitamin D.

Most vegetarians are ovo-lacto vegetarians: They don't eat meat and fish, but they do eat eggs and dairy products. Iron deficiency is the only risk from such a diet. Ovo-lacto vegetarians tend to live longer and develop fewer chronic disabling conditions than people who eat meat. However, their better health may also be a result of their abstention from alcohol and tobacco and their tendency to exercise regularly. Vegetarians who consume no animal products (vegans) are at risk of developing deficiencies of vitamin B12. Oriental-style and other fermented foods, such as fish sauce, can provide vitamin B12.

Many fad diets claim to enhance well-being or reduce weight. However, highly restrictive diets are nutritionally unsound: these diets have resulted in deficiencies of vitamins, minerals, and proteins; in disorders affecting the heart, kidneys, and metabolism; and even in some deaths. Very low calorie diets (fewer than 400 calories a day) can't sustain health for long.

Addiction to alcohol or drugs can disrupt a person's lifestyle to the point that adequate nourishment is neglected and the absorption and metabolism of nutrients are impaired.

Alcoholism is the most common form of drug addiction, with serious effects on nutritional status. Consumed in large amounts, alcohol is a poison that damages tissue, particularly in the gastrointestinal tract, liver, pancreas, and nervous system (including the brain). People who drink beer and continue to consume food may gain weight, but people who consume a fifth of hard liquor daily tend to lose weight and become undernourished. Alcoholism is the most common cause of vitamin B1 (thiamine) deficiency in the United States and may also lead to deficiencies of magnesium, zinc, and other vitamins.

Administration of Nutrients

When nutrients can't be given by mouth, they may be given through a tube (tube feeding) inserted into the gastrointestinal tract (enteral nutrition), or they may be given intravenously (parenteral nutrition). These methods may be used to feed people who are unwilling or unable to eat or who can't digest and absorb nutrients.

Tube Feeding

Tube feeding is used in various situations, including recovery from burns and inflammatory bowel disease. A thin plastic feeding tube (a nasogastric tube) is passed through the nose and gently down the throat until it reaches the stomach or small intestine. Although the insertion of this tube is mildly uncomfortable, most people have little discomfort once it's in place. If tube feeding must be used for a long time, the tube can be placed directly into the stomach or small intestine through a small incision in the abdominal wall.

The solutions used in tube feeding contain all the nutrients a person needs, including proteins, carbohydrates, fats, vitamins, and trace minerals. Fats supply 2 to 45 percent of the total calories.

Problems with tube feeding are uncommon and rarely serious. Some people have diarrhea and abdominal discomfort. The esophagus can become irritated and inflamed by the nasogastric tube. Inhaling (aspirating) food into the lungs, a serious but rare complication, can be prevented by elevating the head of the bed to decrease regurgitation and by giving the solution slowly.

Intravenous Feeding

Intravenous feeding is used when people can't receive adequate nourishment through a nasogastric tube. For instance, people who are severely malnourished and need to undergo surgery, radiation therapy, or chemotherapy or people who have severe burns, paralysis of the gastrointestinal tract, or persistent diarrhea or vomiting may be fed intravenously.

Intravenous feeding can supply part of a person's nutritional requirements or all of them (total parenteral nutrition). A number of solutions are available, and they can be modified for people who have kidney or liver disease. Total parenteral nutrition requires a larger intravenous tube (catheter) than those normally used for intravenous fluids. Consequently, a larger vein, such as the subclavian vein located approximately under the collarbone, is used.

A person receiving total parenteral nutrition is closely monitored for changes in weight and urine output and for signs of infection. If the blood levels of glucose become too high, insulin may be added to the solution. Infection is a constant risk because the catheter is usually left in place for a long time and the feeding solutions that pass through it have a high content of glucose—a substance in which bacteria can grow easily.

Total parenteral nutrition can cause other complications. The liver may enlarge if too many calories, particularly from fats, are consumed. The excess fat in the veins may also cause backaches, fever, chills, nausea, and a low platelet count. However, these problems occur in less than 3 percent of the people receiving total parenteral nutrition. Long-term total parenteral nutrition may produce bone pain.

Starvation

How Starvation Affects Body Systems

System	Effects
Digestive system	Low acid production by the stomach Frequent, often fatal diarrhea
Cardiovascular system	

(heart and blood vessels) Reduced heart size, reduced amount of blood pumped, slow heart rate, and low blood pressure

Ultimately, heart failure

Respiratory system Slow breathing, reduced lung capacity

Ultimately, respiratory failure

Reproductive system Reduced size of ovaries in women and testes in men

Loss of sex drive (libido)

Cessation of menstrual periods

Nervous system Apathy and irritability, although intellect remains intact
Muscular system Low capacity for exercise or work because of reduced muscle size and strength
Hematologic system (blood) Anemia
Metabolic system Low body temperature (hypothermia) frequently contributing to death Fluid accumulation in the skin, resulting mainly from disappearance of fat under the skin
Immune system Impaired ability to fight infections and repair wounds

Starvation may result from fasting, famine, anorexia nervosa, severe gastrointestinal disease, stroke, or coma. The body resists starvation by breaking down its own tissues and using them as a source of calories—much like burning the furniture to keep a house warm. As a result, internal organs and muscle are progressively damaged, and body fat (adipose tissue) nearly disappears.

Adults can lose up to half of their body weight, and children can lose even more. Proportional weight loss is greatest in the liver and intestines, moderate in the heart and kidney, and least in the nervous system. The most obvious signs of emaciation are wasting in areas where the body normally stores fat, reduced muscle size, and protruding bones. The skin becomes thin, dry, inelastic, pale, and cold. The hair, which becomes dry and sparse, falls out easily. Most body systems are affected. Total starvation is fatal in 8 to 12 weeks.

Treatment

Restoring food intake to normal amounts requires a considerable amount of time, depending on how long a person has been without food and how severely the body is affected. The gastrointestinal tract shrinks during starvation and can't accommodate a normal diet all at once. Liquids such as juice, milk, broth, and clear soup are recommended for those who can take food by mouth. After a few days of liquids, a solid diet can be started and increased gradually to 5,000 or more calories a day. Usually, bland foods are recommended, given in small portions at frequent intervals to avoid diarrhea. A person should gain 3 to 4 pounds a week until a normal weight is reached. Some people need to be fed through a nasogastric tube at first. Intravenous feeding may be needed if malabsorption and diarrhea persist.

Protein-Energy Malnutrition

Between the extremes of starvation and adequate nutrition, there are various degrees of inadequate nutrition, such as protein-energy malnutrition, the leading cause of death in children of developing countries. Protein-energy malnutrition is caused by an inadequate consumption of calories, resulting in a deficiency of proteins and micronutrients (nutrients required in small quantities, such as vitamins and trace minerals). Rapid growth, an infection, an injury, or a chronic debilitating disease can increase the need for nutrients, particularly in infants and young children who are already malnourished.

Symptoms

There are three types of protein-energy malnutrition: dry (a person is thin and dehydrated), wet (a person is puffy because of fluid retention), and an intermediate type between the two extremes.

The dry type, called marasmus, results from almost total starvation. A child who has marasmus consumes very little food, often because the mother is unable to breastfeed, and is very thin from the loss of both muscle and body fat.

Almost invariably, an infection develops. If the child is injured or if the infection becomes widespread, the prognosis is worse and the child's life is jeopardized.

The wet type is called kwashiorkor, an African word meaning "first child-second child." It comes from the observation that the first child develops kwashiorkor when the second child is born and replaces the first child at the mother's breast. The weaned first child is fed a thin gruel that's low in nutritional quality compared with mother's milk, so the child does not thrive. The protein deficiency in kwashiorkor is usually more significant than the calorie (energy) deficiency, resulting in fluid retention (edema), skin disease, and discoloration of the hair. Because children develop kwashiorkor after they are weaned, they are usually older than those who have marasmus.

The intermediate type of protein-energy malnutrition is called marasmic kwashiorkor. Children with this type retain some fluid and have more body fat than those who have marasmus.

Kwashiorkor is less common than marasmus and usually occurs as marasmic kwashiorkor. It tends to be confined to parts of the world (rural Africa, the Caribbean, the Pacific islands, and Southeast Asia) where staples and foods used to wean babies—such as yams, cassava, rice, sweet potatoes, and green bananas—are protein-deficient and excessively starchy.

In marasmus, as in starvation, the body breaks down its own tissues to use as calories. Carbohydrates stored in the liver are depleted, proteins in muscle are broken down to synthesize new proteins, and stored fat is broken down to produce calories. As a result, the entire body shrinks.

In kwashiorkor, the body is less able to synthesize new proteins. Consequently, blood levels of proteins decrease, causing fluids to accumulate in the arms and legs as edema. Cholesterol levels also decrease and an enlarged fatty liver (excessive accumulation of fat inside the liver cells) develops. The protein deficiency impairs body growth, immunity, the ability to repair damaged tissues, and the production of enzymes and hormones. In marasmus and kwashiorkor, diarrhea is common.

Behavioral development may be markedly slow in the severely malnourished child, and mental retardation may occur. Usually, an infant who has marasmus is affected more severely than an older child who has kwashiorkor.

Treatment

An infant who has protein-energy malnutrition is usually given intravenous feedings during the first 24 to 48 hours after hospitalization. Because such infants invariably have serious infections, an antibiotic is usually included in the intravenous fluids. A milk-based formula is given by mouth as soon as it can be tolerated. The amount of calories given is gradually increased, so that an infant who weighed 13 to 17 pounds when admitted to the hospital gains about 7 pounds over 12 weeks.

Prognosis

Up to 40 percent of the children who have protein-energy malnutrition die. Death during the first days of treatment is usually caused by an electrolyte imbalance, an infection, an abnormally low body temperature (hypothermia), or heart failure. Stupor (semiconsciousness), jaundice, tiny skin hemorrhages, a low sodium level in the blood, and persistent diarrhea are ominous signs. The disappearance of apathy, edema, and lack of appetite is a favorable sign. Recovery is more rapid from kwashiorkor than from marasmus.

The long-term effects of malnutrition in childhood are unknown. When children are adequately treated, the liver and immune system recover completely. However, in some children, the absorption of nutrients in the intestine remains impaired. The degree of mental impairment is related to how long a child was malnourished, how severe the malnutrition was, and at what age it began. A mild degree of mental retardation may persist into school age and possibly beyond.

High Energy Diets

The most efficient strategy to adopt for any exercise is a gradual build -up over several weeks. All the body systems need to be brought to a state of fitness gradually, not just the muscles. There is no need to increase protein intake to build muscle, most of the protein that you eat will simply be destroyed, putting an extra load on the kidneys.

Keep to a breakfast of starch and fruit (without added sugar) and a lunch of starch and vegetables (without too much added fats) and a single protein meal a day.

If you find your appetite increasing with the extra exercise, add to the starch in your meals, not the protein and not extra fat. If you are to engage in prolonged heavy exercise, such as hard manual labour for more than 8 hours each day, you may even require three starch based meals a day plus the one protein meal. But do resist the temptation to cover the starch with fat or sugar.

For intensive occasional exercise the body is dependent on mobilising reserves already in place rather than deriving them from food immediately before or during the exercise. Training over several weeks ensures that this mobilisation of reserves takes place efficiently and is less likely to cause the highs and lows of blood sugar that result from high sugar and fat diets. Any food remaining in the stomach will reduce the body's capacity to participate in intensive exercise. Do not eat a fatty meal any closer than 4 hours before vigorous exercise. A protein meal requires at least two hours for digestion before starting vigorous exercise and a starch meal one hour.

The food combining diet combined with proper training results in a person who is much fitter and able to enjoy all sporting activities

Diets for Different stages of life

Pregnancy

The food combining diet is ideal for pregnancy because it returns natural control of diet to the appetite mechanism, and allows the natural development of pregnancy, with its hormonal and physical changes.

Resist all cravings that take you outside the food combining diet, but ensure that your diet is as broad as possible. Eat one protein meal every day, and fill up at starch and vegetable meals if you are still hungry.

You are unlikely to put on excess weight while following the food combining diet and maintaining your regular exercise.

You should maintain a higher intake of fat, particularly from oil fish, and dairy fat - cream and butter in moderation. It may be wise to avoid processed fats such as margarines and low fat spreads until the health effects of these are clearer.

Pregnant women should not eat liver because the high vitamin A levels can be toxic.

Breast feeding

Human mother's milk is ideal for human babies. The nutrients are produced in the right quantities and in the right form for the human baby to absorb. Mother's milk also provides antibodies which help protect against infection, it is at the right temperature and at the right concentration. There is not the same risk of infection in equipment or contaminated water supplies. Ideally a mother should breast-feed for at least 6 months.

In a very few cases proteins from food are transported intact into the mothers milk can cause a reaction in the baby. A baby with the coeliac condition may react to gluten from wheat in the mother's diet. Others may react to protein from cow's milk, and, very rarely, to protein from nuts.

A breast-feeding mother should ensure she has a diet rich in magnesium. Good

- sources are nuts, raisins and sultanas, banana, soya products. If she eats two meals based on starch and fruit or vegetables and one protein meal each day, she should not lack any nutrients.
- Formula milks based on modified cows milk must be made up to the exact concentration. A baby's kidneys can be immature and unable to excrete the waste products if there is insufficient liquid in the diet.
- Unmodified cow's milk contains too much phosphorus (as phosphates) for human infants and the calcium can be bonded to the fat and not be properly absorbed. This can result in low blood calcium levels and a risk of muscular spasms. Cow's milk is also particularly low in copper and iron.

- Solid foods should not be introduced before 4 months old and wheat should be avoided until the infant is 9 months to a year old.
- Start by introducing a puree of fruit or vegetables, served cold or just warm, after the milk feed. This can be mashed, ripe banana, apple, pear, or a puree of carrots, potatoes, leeks, cauliflower, parsnips or brown rice. The vegetables should be steamed until cooked with the minimum of water, and freshly prepared for each meal. Keep the meals simple, do not mix all the flavours together, and allow the young child time to taste and play with the new sensation of food.
- Avoid giving the young child any highly flavoured or spiced food, and do not add salt or sugar when cooking or making the puree. Salt should not be added to infant diets as they cannot excrete the excess. Avoid also manufactured sauces and spreads such as tomato sauce which have a very high salt and sugar content.
- When the young child starts to make chewing movements, small soft lumps of food can be included, but not hard foods like peanuts on which the child may choke.
- A stick of carrot or apple should be given for the child to chew on, rather than a rusk.
- Young children between the ages of 9 months and 3 ½ years often absorb iron poorly from their food. Separating starch meals from protein meals should greatly improve iron uptake.

Protein meals for the infant can include cooked egg yolk, and very finely minced or shredded meat. A very small amount of easily digested pulses such as lentils can be included, but avoid the hard-to-digest kidney beans and soya beans.

Toddlers to school age

Young children need concentrated sources of energy in their food. Whole milk rather than reduced fat milk should be given to children aged 1 to 2 years, and those under 5 years should not be given skimmed milk.

From the age of 1 year most children can eat a very similar diet to adults. You should still not add salt or extra sugar to their food.

Try to base their meals on a breakfast of starch and fruit, a lunch of starch and vegetables, and an evening meal of protein and vegetables.

Do not feed them added fibre or high fibre cereals. The extra fibre will fill them up without nourishing them, and will interfere with the uptake of minerals from their food. Whole grain rice, whole-meal bread, potatoes in their skins and fresh fruit and vegetables will provide plenty of fibre.

Food should not be smothered in extra fat, but neither should it be removed from their diet. It is still an important source of energy and fat soluble vitamins

Child Diet

Children who are active and growing rapidly need more nutrients in proportion to their body size than most adults. They have large appetites because they need the extra food. Resist the temptation to let them fill up on biscuits, sweets, crisps, pastry, chips and soft drinks, but encourage them to eat a broad range of fresh fruit and vegetables. The same advice about not adding extra fibre still applies. A good diet will provide more than enough fibre. Try and follow the same pattern of meals as the younger children with starch and fruit for breakfast, starch and vegetables for lunch, and protein, vegetables and fruit for an evening meal.

Packed lunches can easily be based on bread and butter, starch spreads and fresh fruit. Children should always be encouraged to select what they want from a small range of choices, and prepare their own packed meal.

As the school child becomes an adolescent it is still important to encourage good, well balanced eating habits and to encourage healthy exercise. There is increasing evidence that adolescents require this exercise in order to lay down the muscle and bone structure that will carry them through their adult lives.

A girl who becomes pregnant before reaching full maturity is particularly at risk of suffering nutritional deficiencies, as her own body's resources are robbed to provide the nutrients for the baby.

Adult Diets

The average diet is too high in protein, fats and sugar, too highly processed and refined, and too salt! It totally disrupts the natural mechanisms that tell us when we have eaten enough!

A healthy adult diet derives most of its energy from starchy foods, fruit and vegetables, with sufficient protein to provide for growth and repair of tissue.

The appetite mechanisms work on starch meals and they work on protein meals to ensure the delicate balance between the food we need and the food we eat. Unfortunately for eaters of the average diet, the appetite mechanisms do not work on the fat content of refined and processed foods. Even a small imbalance can result in a steady increase in weight and the laying down of body fat. It can also result in the eating disorders of anorexia and bulimia.

If you follow the food-combining rules of separating starch and protein meals, and not adding extra fats and sugar to the diet, the natural appetite mechanisms can return to control how much we eat, without the need for us to make a deliberate effort to control body weight.

Some energy is needed just to stay alive. A sleeping man requires 0.3 MJ/hour just to maintain the life processes and any waking activity that allows the body to rest completely uses slightly more energy. Sitting up at a desk to work will use 0.42MJ/hour. Light domestic work, washing and dressing, about 0.75MJ/hour. Active physical work in carrying loads and using shovels or other manual labour can rise to 1MJ/hour. Similar energy levels are required by sports activities but the particularly high energy requirements of games such as squash at 2MJ/hour can only be sustained for a short time.

A lighter and fitter person will require slightly less energy for the same amount of exercise and, on average, a woman requires slightly less energy than a man for the same work.

Acids

Acids such as hydrochloric acid, nitric acid or sulphuric acid are strong acids. A molecule of hydrochloric acid consists of one negative ion of chlorine and one positive ion of hydrogen. In water, the ions separate completely and can react quickly and strongly with other ions in solution.

pH is the measure of the hydrogen ion concentration in a solution. A pH of 1 is a strong acid with many hydrogen ions. A pH of 14 has few hydrogen ions and is a strong alkali. A ph of 7 is a neutral solution.

Acids such as citric acid or ethanoic acid (vinegar) are weak acids. Although molecules of these acids still contain positive hydrogen ions, they do not separate completely in water.

Substances that can neutralise acids are called bases. If a base will also dissolve in water it is called an alkali.

Alkalis such as sodium hydroxide and potassium hydroxide are strong alkalis. A molecule of sodium hydroxide consists of one positive sodium ion and one negative hydroxide ion (OH-). In water the ions separate completely.

Alkalis such as sodium hydrogencarbonate (bicarbonate of soda) and ammonium hydroxide are weak alkalis. The hydroxide ions do not separate completely in water.

Calcium carbonate is a base. It is not soluble in water, but will react to neutralise an acid and to release carbon dioxide gas.

Blood, lymph and the fluids that bathe our cells must stay within a very narrow pH. Any tendency to change has to be counteracted straight away. The body produces substances called buffers, which react with any acid or alkali to maintain a constant pH. The most important buffer is sodium hydrogencarbonate.

The mineral ions of sodium, calcium and potassium used to be called the 'alkaline earth elements' because they form the positive ions of strong alkalis. If food containing these elements is burnt in oxygen and the ash dissolved in water, an alkali is obtained.

Dr Hay's references to alkaline foods are simply an injunction to eat foods that have useful levels of calcium and potassium salts: to eat plenty of fresh fruit and vegetables every day!

Protein in the diet which is not needed for growth or repair of tissue has to be destroyed. The amino acids are converted into urea and uric acid which have to pass into the bloodstream to be eliminated by the kidney. A high protein diet results in the production of excess acid which can put the acid / alkali balance under strain, as well as causing problems for the kidney which has to eliminate the acid.

Carbohydrates are compounds of carbon, hydrogen and oxygen.

Fats are compounds of fatty acids and glycerol, again built from carbon, hydrogen and oxygen, but with less oxygen than the carbohydrates. This makes them a more compact form of energy.

Proteins all contain nitrogen in addition to the carbon, hydrogen and oxygen. They form the tissues which make living things work and control the processes within the cells.

Carbohydrates

Most of our food starts off in the green leaves of plants, where the energy from sunlight is trapped. This energy is then used to join a molecule of water to a molecule of carbon dioxide to form a simple sugar. If the plant wants this energy for some other purpose it can split the simple sugar and add oxygen to the parts, to reform water and carbon dioxide. The energy is then used to keep all the living processes in the cell going.

Unfortunately for the plant, simple sugars are not easily stored in its cells, because they dissolve in water. To overcome this problem, the plant joins two simple sugars together to make a slightly larger sugar molecule, but then joins these in long chains to make starch. These starch molecules are an excellent way of storing the sun's energy and are the main source of energy in food..

Starches are a good way of storing energy, but for some purposes take up too much space. The same energy can be stored in a small space if the molecules are altered to produce oils and fats. Plants will often manufacture oils to store energy for seeds and nuts.

Starches and sugars are known as carbohydrates, because they only contain the elements carbon, hydrogen and oxygen.

Starches are also known as polysaccharides - compounds built of many sugar molecules. Non-starch polysaccharides are known collectively as dietary fibre.

Sugars

Monosaccharides (single sugars) such as glucose and fructose are the simplest sugars. The more complex sugars and starches are broken down into these during digestion.

Disaccharides (two sugars) such as sucrose, maltose and lactose are formed of two simple sugar molecules linked together.

Many people cannot digest lactose (milk sugar) as they grow older.

Sugars inside fruit, or formed by the digestion of starch are released slowly from food and absorbed steadily by the blood-stream. Sugars added to food or drinks are digested much more quickly and surges of sugar entering the bloodstream can cause fluctuations in blood sugar levels that have a harmful effect on health.

Non-sugar sweeteners provide a sweet alternative to sugar, but since they are all highly processed, and not a useful part of the diet, are best avoided.

Starch

Polysaccharides are long chains of glucose molecules which are formed into granules in the storage organs of plants. They are insoluble in water and in this form are indigestible. When heated with water, the starch absorbs the water, swells and gelatinises and can then be broken down by the digestive system. If the processing takes place without water, part of the starch remains indigestible. This happens in the production of some breakfast cereals.

Dietary Fibre consists of the cellulose cell walls and the pectins and gums that cannot be digested by the human system (although they can be digested by a cow). Dietary fibre helps the correct passage of food through the digestive system. A diet rich in fresh fruit and vegetables will provide sufficient fibre. Excess fibre can trap minerals such as calcium, iron, copper and zinc. Wheat fibre is also abrasive and in excess can scratch the lining of the digestive system.

Fats are combinations of fatty acids and glycerol. A mixture of all types of fatty acids is needed for normal health.

Saturated fats

These have their carbon chain saturated with hydrogen atoms. These are stable fats and keep well. Palmitic acid and stearic acid form butter, lard, suet and cocoa butter. Myristic acid forms part of butter and coconut oil.

Unsaturated fats

If hydrogen atoms are missing from the carbon chain, the carbon atoms double-bond to each other instead. Mono-unsaturated fats have a single double-bond, but poly-unsaturated fats have more double-bonds. These double bonds are more reactive and the fat easily combines with oxygen from the air to go rancid.

We need a range of fats in our diet.

Oleic acid forms 60% -70% of olive oil and rapeseed oil.

Linoleic acid is found in seed oils such as maize, soya and sunflower.

Linolenic occurs in vegetable oils in small amounts.

Arachidonic acid only occurs in animal fats, but it can be formed from linoleic acid.

Decosahexaenoic acid is found in oily fish.

The double bonds in natural unsaturated fats are normally in the 'cis' position. This is the natural structure that are body expects. When margarine is being manufactured, some of these bonds are changed into the 'trans' position. These are totally alien to our bodies. These trans fats may increase levels of blood cholesterol and increase the risk of heart disease

All living things need to be able to do far more than simply store energy. Almost all living things are built from vast collections of cells, and cells have to be able to grow. They also move themselves or materials within the cells, exchange messages with other cells, and most are able to reproduce. Eventually all cells die.

In order to carry out these important life processes, a cell needs many different proteins.

Proteins are large, complex molecules built from over twenty different amino acids to form long, complex chains of hundreds or thousands of amino acid units. When a plant cell is producing protein, it first uses the energy of sunlight to join nitrogenous compounds and sugar to make amino acids. Then it joins these amino acids in a very precise way, in long chains. These chains curl up into complicated 3D shapes. A protein has to have the right amino acids in the correct order. Just as each récipe in this book is built from 26 letters of the alphabet, but they must all be in the right order if the recipe is to make sense, and work. Some of these amino acids are common in plants, but some are rare.

We, like most other animals, are unable to manufacture these amino acids from their elements. We have to eat them all as protein in food, then break them down into their building blocks, amino acids.

We cannot simply use plant protein, or other animal protein. We have to make human protein.

Amino acids are needed to produce the proteins that make the walls of human or animal cells, as well as most of the complicated structures within every cell. Amino acids are needed to form the protein that is the part of a muscle cell that contracts, as well as the tough surface of a skin cell. Proteins also form the fine tendrils of nerve cells.

Proteins also control all the processes that take place in every cell to keep us alive. These proteins are called enzymes. Enzymes control all the processes that keep us alive, both inside cells, and outside cells in our digestive system.

There are only 20 different amino acids but they can be arranged in an infinite number of ways. It is the sequence of amino acids in the chain, and the way they cause the chain to twist and fold, that determine the function of the protein. In digestion, the protein chain is split into the. individual amino acids. These are then reassembled in our cells to form the wide variety of human protein.

Indispensable amino acids must be obtained from the food that we eat.

These are Isoleucine, Leucine, Lysine, Methionine, Phenylalanine, Threonine, Tryptophan, Valine, Histidine is also essential in the diet of young children.

The following amino acids are also essential, but they can be manufactured inside our own bodies by breaking down and re-assembling other amino acids.

Alanine, Arginine, Aspartic acid, Asparagine, Cysteine, Glutamic acid, Glutamine, Glycine, Proline, Serine, Tyrosine.

The amino acids in animal proteins from meat, fish, milk, cheese and eggs match closely that required by humans. Plant proteins often have a marked imbalance of amino acids. Wheat and rice are low in lysine, peas and beans are low in tryptophan and methionine. Mixtures of a broad variety of plant foods will produce a balance of amino acids closer to our requirements. Mixtures of cereals provide the main source of protein for many people.

Surplus protein cannot be stored in our bodies, and if energy is in short supply protein will be broken down as an energy source rather than be used for growth.

If you follow the food combining lifestyle you will get all the vitamins, minerals and trace elements that you require without the need to take any supplements.

Serve green vegetables with a dab of butter or add a dressing of olive oil as this increases the absorption of vitamins by the body. This is because these vitamins are only soluble in oil, not water.

- Vitamin A: retinol is made inside our bodies from beta carotene which gives the orange and yellow colour to fruits and vegetables. Good sources are carrots, sweet potatoes, apricots, mango, yellow fleshed melon, peaches, nectarines, pumpkin, tomato, spinach, watercress and dark green leafy vegetables. We only make as much vitamin A as we need.
- Vitamin A is also found in liver, kidney, cheese, eggs and cod liver oil. Smaller amounts are obtained from yogurt, milk, butter and oily fish such as mackerel and

sardines. If we eat too much liver, we can overdose on vitamin A, and suffer joint pains until we have used up the excess. One meal of liver per week provides a good source of iron without excess vitamin A. Pregnant women should not eat liver as the excess vitamin A can damage the foetus.

- Vitamin A is important for the care of the eyes, and for the immune system to fight off infection. It is essential for normal growth and repair of tissues. It is also important in reducing the risk of cancer and heart disease.
- Vitamin B1: thiamine is needed to release the energy from food. Good sources are potatoes, wholegrain cereals, green vegetables, pulses, nuts and sunflower seeds. Diets high in refined starch can suffer from B1 deficiency.
- Vitamin B2: riboflavine is needed to release the energy from food. Good sources are liver, meat, milk and cheese.
- Vitamin B3 (PP): niacin or nicotinic acid, is needed to release the energy from food. Good sources are peas and beans, liver, meat and wholegrain cereals. This vitamin in maize is unavailable unless treated with alkali. The body can make niacin from the tryptophan present in eggs.
- Vitamin B5: pantothenic acid is needed to make energy available to the body's cells. Good sources are egg, liver, kidney, cheese, mushrooms, peanuts and banana.
- Vitamin B6: pyridoxine is needed to make proper use of proteins. Good sources are liver, cereal, pulses and poultry. Supplements are potentially dangerous as an excess can result in nerve damage
- Vitamin B12: cobalamin is essential for the formation of red blood cells. Good sources are meat, milk, cheese and eggs. Vegans are at risk from a characteristic anaemia as B12 does not occur in vegetable food.
- Vitamin B(M): folic acid is also essential for the formation of red blood cells. Good sources are broccoli, spinach, brussels sprouts and other green leafy vegetables, beetroot, broad beans, sweet corn, eggs, liver and whole grain cereals. The Department of Health advises 400ug a day for pregnant women to reduce risk of spina bifida.

- Vitamin B(H): biotin is needed to make energy available from fat. Good sources are liver, kidney, pork, wholegrain cereals, lentils, nuts, cauliflower. It is also produced by bacteria in the large intestine.
- Vitamin C: ascorbic acid is essential to keep our connective tissues healthy and to heal wounds. It is also needed to enable iron to be absorbed from food. Good sources are blackcurrants, cherries, strawberries, kiwi fruit, gooseberries, peppers, guava, oranges, sprouts, cauliflower, potato. Vitamin C is water soluble so cook vegetables by steaming or in a microwave without adding water. Use the water that vegetables are cooked in to make soups or sauces.
- Vitamin D: calciferol helps the body make proper use of calcium in bones and teeth. Good sources are sunlight, oily fish, eggs, butter, yogurt. Too high a vitamin D intake from the food can result in excess calcium being absorbed from the food resulting in damage to the kidneys.
- Vitamin E: tocopherol mops up dangerous chemicals in the bloodstream -100IU a day has been shown to be beneficial. Good sources are eggs, butter, vegetable oil, oily fish, almonds, avocado, pine kernels, wholegrain cereals and sunflower seeds.
- Vitamin F: linoleic and alpha linolenic acids. These are known to be essential for the correct functioning of cell membranes. Good sources are vegetable oils.

Almost all minerals are found in the human body and 15 of them are known to be essential. They will be absorbed in the right amounts in a properly balanced and combined diet, but most of the trace elements and iron and zinc are poisonous if extra is eaten.

- Potassium is essential to maintain the right balance of acids and alkalis in the body. It is needed in order to excrete excess acid. Low levels of potassium in the diet are linked to high blood pressure and an increased risk of stroke. Good sources are tomato, strawberries, banana, other fruit, yogurt, cheese, potatoes, soya products, whole grain cereals, nuts, black treacle. Deficiency is unlikely to occur on the diet described by this book unless diuretics or purgatives are taken, or in cases of diarrhoea linked to malnutrition.

- Iron is needed for the production of red blood cells, for muscle tissue and for handling oxygen in many other cells. Good sources are liver, red meat, fish, raisins and sultanas, green vegetables. Tannins from tea and an excess of wheat fibre can reduce the uptake of iron.
- Magnesium for healthy bones, nerves and muscle. Good sources are nuts, raisins and sultanas, banana, soya products. Deficiency is rare except in cases of severe diarrhoea.
- Zinc is needed for the growth of all healthy tissue, muscle and bone and for the healing of wounds. Good sources are red meat, liver, hard cheese but zinc uptake is reduced if cereal fibre is eaten at the same time, Wholegrain cereals also contain useful levels of zinc.
- Phosphorus is an important part of all healthy cells, especially bones and teeth. Good sources are meat and other proteins.
- Calcium is needed for healthy bones and teeth. Good sources are milk and cheese, yogurt, wholegrain cereals, pulses, vegetables, raisins and sultanas. Vitamin D is essential for the correct uptake of calcium from the diet. Wheat fibre also reduces calcium uptake.
- Sodium and chloride are both essential elements for muscle and nerve activity. A diet rich in processed foods is likely to contain excessively high sodium levels and increase the risk of high blood pressure.

These are the elements that are essential for the body to work, but needed only in very small amounts.

- Chromium is needed for insulin production.
- Good sources are shellfish, brewers yeast, beef, chicken, whole grain cereals, nuts and black treacle.
- Copper is used in the manufacture of red blood cells and many enzymes.
- Good sources are shellfish, kidney, whole grain cereals, liver, green vegetables, fish.
- Iodine is needed to make thyroid hormones and for the development of the nervous system.
- Good sources are fish, shell fish, milk, whole grain cereals, but vegans may be prone to low iodine levels.
- Selenium is important for some enzymes.
- Good sources are liver, meat, fish, whole grain cereals.
- Manganese is needed for many enzymes to operate.

- Cereals and nuts are good sources

The digestive system

Our digestive system evolved over many millions of years to match the lifestyle of our ancestors, who hunted for meat or fish, and gathered seeds, fruits, roots and berries.

The change in our ancestors' way of life to an agricultural and then industrial lifestyle has been so quick that the power of evolution to match the way our body works to the way we live has not yet had time to operate. We still have a digestive system designed to match millions of years of a hunter-gatherer existence.

Our bodies are designed to work their best using a variety of different types of food.

Animals like the cow, which evolved to eat only vegetable food, have developed a series of pouches, or extra stomachs, to separate one meal from the next. As digestion progresses food is moved from one to the next, or even brought back to the mouth for a further chew.

Our digestive system is designed to cope in two distinct ways according to whether the food is mostly protein or mostly starch.

The process of making food available for our cells to use starts with cooking. Starches in cereals, pulses and tubers need to be softened and gelatinised by a period of moist cooking before they can be digested. Cellulose cell walls need to be ruptured by the cooking process before the contents are accessible to digestion. Meat fibres also need to be softened to improve their digestibility.

Cooking also destroys the toxins that many plants contain. For example red kidney beans require over-night soaking and then boiling rapidly for ten minutes before they are safe to eat.

Food in the mouth is broken down mechanically and mixed with salivary amylase. The amylase will only start the digestion of starch in a neutral solution. If the food is acid it will not work. If the starch is coated in fat, then digestion of the starch will be limited.

The stomach produces gastric juice in response to the food entering the stomach. About three litres of juice are produced each day. The strong muscular walls mix the food with the gastric juices. The gastric juice contains much more of the enzyme pepsin and more hydrochloric acid when protein enters the stomach. This is a 0.2% to 0.4% solution of acid which is much stronger than acid foods. The acid provides the conditions needed for the digestion of protein as well as destroying most bacteria eaten with the food. A protein meal will remain between 2 - 4 hours in the stomach.

ach to a staA starch and vegetable meal will pass through the stomach very quickly without stimulating the production of large amounts of acid or pepsin.

Fat can bring the digestion in the stomndstill. The contents remain acid for a prolonged period and this can give rise to discomfort.

Small amounts of water, minerals such as sodium chloride, most B vitamins, vitamin C and alcohol are all absorbed directly from the stomach. Simple sugars are also absorbed and if the food contains too much sugar, this can result in a dangerous surge in blood sugar levels.

The semi-liquid partially digested food (chyme) is allowed to move slowly into the small intestine. Here, bile from the liver emulsifies the fats into tiny droplets. An alkaline liquid from the pancreas neutralises the stomach acid. In the neutral solution, the enzyme lipase splits the fats into fatty acids and glycerol, the enzyme amylase splits starch into maltose. The enzymes trypsin and chymotripsin continue to split proteins into short chain peptides and amino acids.

The final stages of digestion take place when the food is in contact with the cells that line the walls of the small intestine. The food molecules are absorbed by the cells and any remaining peptides are split into amino acids, maltose is converted to glucose, sucrose into glucose and fructose, lactose into glucose and galactose. Most of the absorption of digested food takes place through the surface of the small intestine, whose surface area is greatly increased by tiny finger-like projections called villi. Laxatives and excessive fibre interfere with the absorption of food, and phytic acid in wholemeal breakfast cereals can interfere with the uptake of calcium, iron and zinc.

The remaining cellulose and other fibre and indigestible remains now get processed by bacteria in the large intestine. These bacteria form some B-vitamins as well as useful amounts of vitamin K which are absorbed through the walls of the large intestine.

All the products of the digestion of starch and sugars form simple sugars which are carried by the bloodstream directly to the liver. The liver keeps a close control of the level of sugar in the blood, supplying the tissues with a constant level of glucose and storing the surplus as glycogen in the liver and muscles. When the glycogen reserves are full, further surplus sugar is converted into fat for storage.

Fatty acids absorbed by the small intestine do not pass directly into the bloodstream, but are converted back into fats and added to the lymph fluid. This rejoins the bloodstream but bypasses the liver. The fat circulates in the bloodstream and is available as an energy source for the body cells. Fat in the diet is more easily converted into body fat than carbohydrate in the diet.

A protein meal of meat, cheese or eggs, is broken up by the teeth and passed down to the stomach. In response to the arrival of the protein, the stomach lining produces a strong acid, and enzymes which digest protein in acid solution, and a thick sticky mucus to protect the lining of the stomach from attack by its own enzymes. These enzymes snip the long protein molecules in our food into shorter chains and then into individual amino acids.

A meal of protein may take several hours for complete digestion before passing on into the small intestine. Here the stomach acid is neutralised by bile salts from the liver. The pancreas now adds further protein digesting enzymes to complete the digestion of protein and the soup of amino acids is now absorbed through the villi that line the small intestine and are passed on into the blood stream.

A meal of starch is partly digested in the mouth where chewing mixes enzymes in the alkaline saliva with the food. The starch molecule is split into sugar molecules. A starch meal does not stimulate the stomach to produce acid, or protein digesting enzymes, and the food is passed on to the small intestine within an hour. In the small intestine, further enzymes are added in an alkaline solution that complete the breakdown of starches into sugars. These are also absorbed through the villi that line the small intestine and pass into the blood stream.

This system only works efficiently if starch and protein appear as separate meals. The food combining lifestyle puts this scientific knowledge into practice.

If starch is mixed with protein, the enzymes in the stomach are diluted and the stomach feels full for longer because digestion of protein is inefficient. Acid is being produced for every mixed meal, which puts the stomach under stress. The acid has to be neutralised by the bile salts for every meal, which puts the small intestine under stress.

Whole grain cereals contain starch with a little protein. They are digested comparatively slowly, but efficiently by the starch digestion process, but there are enough protein digesting enzymes in the small intestine to ensure the proteins as well as the starches are digested. The sugars that result from the digestion of starch are absorbed by the villi, and passed into the bloodstream for several hours. The liver is able to convert sugars not immediately required into glycogen for storage. If more sugar is absorbed than can be converted into glycogen, the surplus will be changed into fat.

White flour is almost pure starch. It mixes easily with saliva in the mouth and breaks down rapidly into sugars. As soon as the digested starch reaches the small intestine, a huge surge of sugars passes into the bloodstream. Insulin is produced rapidly to control it and the liver is put under stress to process the surplus. The body works flat out to remove the surplus from the bloodstream, and usually overshoots, leaving the bloodstream with too low sugar levels, and the person feeling tired and lacking in energy. These fluctuating blood sugar levels can put the body under too much stress and the system controlling blood sugar starts to break down. The result can be diabetes.

Refined sugar is even worse because it requires no further digestion but enters the bloodstream in a dangerous surge.

Protein is digested to amino acids which are then absorbed into the bloodstream. These amino acids are then absorbed by all cells that require them for growth or the repair of tissue and are built up again into human protein.

All amino acids not needed for growth and repair have to be destroyed. The liver removes the amino group and converts the rest into sugar and then glycogen or fat. The amino group has to be converted into urea which is then removed from the blood by the kidneys.

Both the amino group and urea form an acid solution. Potassium and calcium are needed to neutralise this acid and are lost to the body. Excess protein in the diet puts the liver under stress. The loss of calcium may be made up by removing calcium from the bones and loss of potassium makes it more difficult for the body to balance the acid and alkaline substances in solution. The kidney has to deal with the acid end product of excess protein in the diet and is put under stress.

One protein meal a day provides most of us with all the protein that we need.

Diet & Appetite

Our ancestors for many millions of years ate a diet based on starchy foods, fruit and vegetables, with the occasional meal of protein to provide for growth and repair of tissue. They were rarely exposed to fat in the diet that wasn't closely linked to the plant or animal from which it came. As a result our appetite mechanisms evolved to work on starch meals or on protein meals to ensure the delicate balance between the food we need and the food we eat.

Our ancestors' digestive system evolved to work optimally with either the starch, fruit and vegetables that could be gathered each day, or the protein that was occasionally found as a nest of eggs, or caught. To this day our digestive system works most efficiently when protein and starch meals are kept separate. There have been too few generations of humans since our diets changed for our digestive systems to change to cope well with the mixtures that are now available.

Good Nutrition and Sports

Excess weight aggravates the potential for injury and adds to the strain on the joints . Lack of proper hydration, muscle strength imbalances, lack of strength in the muscles most stressed by your sport, and lack of muscle flexibility are other preconditions for being injury prone. Improper diet may provide inadequate fuel for sports, induce fatigue, and enhance the risk for injury. Let's deal first with weight here.

First, there are 3,500 calories in a pound. Generally, a healthy adult will consume or metabolize 2,900 calories a day without activity. In order to gain weight, you would have to create a calorie surplus of 3,500. One meal where you indulge isn't going to hurt unless you string together 20 indulgences in a row.

Let's do the math. Let's say, you eat one egg sandwich for breakfast (with hash browns), a big hamburger and fries for lunch with an apple pie, and do the same for dinner. Let's also say you wash it down with a six pack. Give or take, you have consumed over 4,000 calories. Let's further assume you didn't feel like exercising, so you only consumed 2,900 calories. For the day, you created a surplus of 1,100 calories. In a week, continuing this eating pattern, you would have created a surplus of 7,700 calories or 2.2 pounds. OK. No problem.

It is a problem, because, if you continue this for a year, you would be a perfect sphere. To do the math, you would gain over 50 pounds. Bombarding your taste buds with the intensity created by a high saturated fat, high salt, and high sugar diet make healthy food taste so bland that it is difficult to escape the captivity of bad food.

The consequence of this excess calorie consumption is either an early coronary, or a commitment to lose weight. Diet fads are a dime a dozen and most of them fail. Celebrity pitchpersons may sell the program, but they won't make it successful beyond the financial aspects for themselves.

Here are the sad facts. Most diets involve calorie deprivation. If you reduce your caloric intake below 1,000 for a period of time (weeks, for example), your body's natural metabolic rate will lower itself and make do with what you give it. When you cease the diet, and return to your normal intake, you will create bigger calorie surplus because it will take the body time for the metabolic rate to rise to meet the higher intake. In the meantime, you will experience the "yo yo", where you gain back more than you lost.

To lose weight, you need to create calorie deficits. The best way to do this is twofold. First, reduce your intake below 2,500 calories, but above 1,800 calories (go much lower and you slow your metabolic rate). Second, stop eating processed foods. This means go to the produce section and get fruits and vegetables. Eat salads, fresh fruit and vegetables. Get your proteins from lean skinless sources like chicken or fish. Additionally, you can get protein from soy beans (Japanese Etemomi beans are great) or mixtures of rice and beans. Most sources of protein are derived from animals and animal by-products and are, therefore, high in saturated fat. During a period where weight loss is a target it is wise to consume non-animal protein sources.

If you are overweight and follow this common sense approach for one month in conjunction with a vigorous exercise program, you will lose weight and feel great. This type of program will make you lean and give you great fuel for your athletic activities.

Here's another two ways to approach nutrition. First, if it comes wrapped in paper or in a box with enticing pictures, it is probably bad for you. Second, don't anticipate food for the way it momentarily titillates your taste buds. Rather, concentrate on how you feel the minute after the momentary titillation of the taste buds subsides. If you do, you will gravitate to carrots, not cake, fruit, not french fries, and pears, not pizza.

If you are moving from a junk diet, it will take a few days to purge your taste buds requirement to be bombarded by high fat, sugar and sodium diets. Soon, you create a taste and yen for fruit and vegetables, at the same time you are getting leaner, and more energetic.

I repeat, focus on how you will feel after you eat, not what it tastes like when you eat. The rest will probably take care of itself.

Food as Fuel

You are what you eat is an old expression that has revitalized currency as the the link between performance and diet continues to be reaffirmed.

Today, the statistics provided on food labels can provide anyone with information on fat, calories, protein, fiber and much more. With both the diet and performance implications of your diet, there are no magic wands, silver bullets, or short cuts to achieve superior results. What you need to know is on the labels. The rest is consistency and discipline.

What are your basic diet requirements? First, you want to achieve an approximate calorie target without obsessing on counting and making your friends crazy. Second you want to achieve an appropriate balance in your diet of roughly 55% carbohydrates, 10% protein and 35% fat, almost exclusively from non-saturated sources. (Saturated fat is in solid form at room tennperatures. You eat fat, you get fat.) These are the recommendations of the American Dietetic Association.

Carbohydrates originate from fruits, vegetables, grains, and processed flours and sugars. Keeping the sugar portion of the diet to a minimum is essential. Refined sugars and chocolates do not create energy, they cause the liver to freak out, followed quickly by weakness. Please avoid this trap. The Snickers ads are appealing, but eating them will hurt your performance.

The body converts simple (candy, fruit, juice, etc.) and complex (pasta, potatoes, cereal, etc.) carbohydrates into glucose, which is burned for quick energy; any extra gets stored in the muscles as glycogen. It's these glycogen stores that the muscles rely on for the extra exertion of athletic competition. Anytime you plan to be physically active for more than an hour, it's going to be harmful to your performance to be on a very high simple carbohydrate diet.

All the glucose is going to burn away, your insulin levels will rise, you'll become weak and sweaty and you'll be in for trouble. A mainstay in the diet for very active people is complex carbohydrates, which provide the energy for sustained activity.

If you're tremendously active—training for marathons or any other endurance sport—physical activity that goes on hour after hour and day after day, fat in the diet is essential. There is no way we can eat that many carbohydrates to keep up with the demands of a hugely active body, so fats can supply a source of energy for extended physical activity. Marathon runners are coming around to this fact.

(If you are a marathon runner, you will need this topic for the injuries to the back, hips, knees and feet that will inevitably follow your participation in this physically destructive sport. If your goal is general fitness and long a long active life of participation, this highly destructive sport simply puts too much strain on the joints.)

Protein is derived from animals and animal by-products. Protein is what comprises the muscles. Cells are constantly dieing and being destroyed. During the day, this cell destruction must be replaced. Lean sources of protein like skinless chicken and fish is recommended over fatty red meats. Protein is also needed since certain vitamins are fat soluble and the lack of these vitamins is unhealthy.

Fat is a product of animals and their by-products, cheeses, milks, cottage cheese, ice cream, etc..

I think the current guidelines are two heavy on the fat, and need real specificity as to the sources of fats, carbohydrates, and protein. Specifically, you could superficially meet these targets with a diet high in sugars, fats, and salts.

If you get your carbs from grains, vegetables and fruits, your protein from lean sources like skinless chicken and fish, and get your fat in unsaturated form you do not need to obsess on scientific precision. If you are not fat, have good energy, and do not fade in your chosen sport, your diet is probably on the mark.

Younger people need more protein to develop muscles. Heavy weight lifters need more protein because of the cell destruction from heavy lifting. As you get older your body needs less

Amino acids are the building blocks of proteins. Despite a lot of hype, amino substitutes appear to be redundant for those with a proper balanced diet.

Football players, being in a sport that emphasizes strength and requires weight training, need to get enough protein to maintain and gain muscle. The long-distance runner needs maximum stores of glycogen to supply him with energy over time. Those involved in lengthy tennis matches or other aerobic activity need to make sure they attend to their nutritional needs for both fuel and cell nutrition before, during, and after their sport.

Myriad supplements exist for which adequate testing and evidence is not available in definitive form. However, it is available in anecdotal form. Creatine is an example. In truth, it will help in strength sports and help one gain more muscle, power and mass. However, it is not a source of energy and does not meet your nutritional requirements. Dehydration and muscle pulls are a frequent product of this supplement.

Fluid intake for athletes are as critical a concern as nutrition. Hydration must be a lifestyle event. The way you eat is not about temporary deprivation followed by rampant excess. Likewise, fluid intake and proper hydration cannot occur just during the sport. You must drink water before, during and after your sport.

Once you are thirsty, it is probably too late to rehydrate on the fly during your event. You can't repair a car at 50 miles per hour, and you can't successfully rehydate after the thirst has set in.

When you are thirsty, you are already 3 % dehydrated and in most sports, this leads to at least a 10 percent decrease in performance ability, if not outright failure.

Hydration is about good old water, not sports drinks. Save your money, drink water.

CHAPTER 2

WEIGHT EVALUATION

For adults and children, different methods are used to find out if weight is about right for height. If you have concerns about your child's body size, talk with your health care provider. Also see the section Encourage healthy weight in children. If you are an adult, follow the directions in INDEX to evaluate your weight in relation to your height, or Body Mass Index (BMI). Not all adults who have a BMI in the range labeled "healthy" are at their most healthy weight. For example, some may have lots of fat and little muscle. A BMI above the healthy range is less healthy for most people; but it may be fine if you have lots of muscle and little fat. The further your BMI is above the healthy range, the higher your weight-related risk. If your BMI is above the healthy range, you may benefit from weight loss, especially if you have other health risk factors (see INDEX 2).

BMI's slightly below the healthy range may still be healthy unless they result from illness. If your BMI is below the healthy range, you may have increased risk of menstrual irregularity, infertility, and osteoporosis. If you lose weight suddenly or for unknown reasons, see a health care provider. Unexplained weight loss may be an early clue to a health problem.

Keep track of your weight and your waist measurement, and take action if either of them increases. If your BMI is greater than 25, or even if it is in the "healthy" range, at least try to avoid further weight gain. If your waist measurement increases, you are probably gaining fat. If so, take steps to eat fewer calories and become more active.

INDEX 1

HOW TO EVALUATE YOUR WEIGHT (ADULTS)

1. Weigh yourself and have your height measured. Find your BMI category in figure 1. The higher your BMI category, the greater the risk for health problems.
2. Measure around your waist, just above your hip bones, while standing. Health risks increase as waist

measurement increases, particularly if waist is greater than 35 inches for women or 40 inches for men. Excess abdominal fat may place you at greater risk of health problems, even if your BMI is about right.

3. Use INDEX 2 to find out how many other risk factors you have. The higher your BMI and waist measurement, and the more risk factors you have from INDEX 2, the more you are likely to benefit from weight loss.

NOTE: Weight loss is usúally not advisable for pregnant women.

FIND OUT YOUR OTHER RISK FACTORS FOR CHRONIC DISEASE

The more of these risk factors you have, the more you are likely to benefit from weight loss if you are overweight or obese.

- Do you have a personal or family history of heart disease?
- Are you a male older than 45 years or a postmenopausal female?
- Do you smoke cigarettes?
- Do you have a sedentary lifestyle?
- Has your doctor told you that you have
- high blood pressure?
- abnormal blood lipids (high LDL cholesterol, low HDL cholesterol, high triglycerides)?
- diabetes?

Manage your weight

Our genes affect our tendency to gain weight. A tendency to gain weight is increased when food is plentiful and when we use equipment and vehicles to save time and energy. However, it is possible to manage your weight through balancing the calories you eat with your physical activity choices.

To make it easier to manage your weight, make long-term changes in your eating behavior and physical activity. To do this, build a healthy base and make sensible choices. Choose a healthful assortment of foods that includes vegetables, fruits, grains (especially whole grains), skim milk, and fish, lean meat, poultry, or beans. Choose foods that are low in fat and added sugars most of the time (see section Choose Sensibly). Whatever the food, eat a sensible portion size (see INDEX 3).

Try to be more active throughout the day. The physical activity guideline (see section Be Physically Active Each Day) recommends that all adults get at least 30 minutes of moderate physical activity most or preferably all days of the week. To maintain a healthy weight after weight loss, adults will likely need to do more than 30 minutes of moderate physical activity daily. Over time, even a small decrease in calories eaten and a small increase in physical activity can keep you from gaining weight or help you lose weight.

INDEX 3

CHOOSE SENSIBLE PORTION SIZES

Control portion size. See guideline "Let the Pyramid guide your food choices" for sensible sizes and numbers of servings.

- If you're eating out, choose small portion sizes, share an entree with a friend, or take part of the food home (if you can chill it right away).
- Check product labels to learn how much food is considered to be a serving, and how many calories, grams of fat, and so forth are in the food. Many items sold as single portions actually provide 2 servings or more. Examples include a 20-ounce container of soft drink, a 12-ounce steak, a 3-ounce bag of chips, and a large bagel.
- Be especially careful to limit portion size of foods high in calories, such as cookies, cakes, other sweets, French fries, and fats, oils, and spreads.

The carbohydrates, fats, and proteins in food supply energy, which is measured in calories. High-fat foods contain more calories than the same amount of other foods, so they can make it difficult for you to avoid excess calories. However, low fat doesn't always mean low calorie. Sometimes extra sugars are added to low-fat muffins or desserts, for example, and they may be just as high in calories.

Your pattern of eating may be important. Snacks and meals eaten away from home provide a large part of daily calories for many people. Choose them wisely. Try fruits, vegetables, whole grain foods, or a cup of low-fat milk or yogurt for a snack. When eating out, choose small portions of foods. If you choose fish, poultry, or lean meat, ask that it be grilled rather than fried.

Like younger adults, overweight and obese older adults may improve their health by losing weight. The guidance of a health care provider is recommended, especially for obese children and older adults. Since older people tend to lose muscle mass, regular physical activity is a valuable part of a weight-loss plan. Building or maintaining muscle helps keep older adults active and reduces their risk of falls and fractures. Staying active throughout your adult years helps maintain muscle mass and bone strength for your later years.

If you need to lose weight, do so gradually

If you are overweight, loss of 5 to 15 percent of your body weight may improve your health, ability to function, and quality of life. Aim to lose about 10 percent of your weight over about 6 months. This would be 20 pounds of weight loss for someone who weighs 200 pounds. Loss of ½ to 2 pounds per week is usually safe. Even if you have regained weight in the past, it's worthwhile to try again.

Encourage healthy weight in children

Children need enough food for proper growth, but too many calories and too little physical activity lead to overweight. The number of overweight U.S. children has risen dramatically in recent years. Encourage healthy weight by offering children grain products; vegetables and fruits; low-fat dairy products; and beans, lean meat, poultry, fish, or nuts—and let them see you enjoy eating the same foods. Let the child decide how much of these foods to eat. Offer only small amounts of food high in fat or added sugars. Encourage children to take part in vigorous activities (and join them whenever possible). Limit the time they spend in sedentary activities like watching television or playing computer or video games.

Help children to develop healthy eating habits. Make small changes. For example, serve low-fat milk rather than whole milk and offer one cookie instead of two. Since children still need to grow, weight loss is not recommended unless guided by a health care provider.

Serious eating disorders

Frequent binge eating, with or without periods of food restriction, may be a sign of a serious eating disorder. Other signs of eating disorders include preoccupation with body weight or food (or both—regardless of body weight), dramatic weight loss, excessive exercise, self-induced vomiting, and the abuse of laxatives. Seek help from a health care provider if any of these apply to you, a family member, or a friend.

Aim for a healthy weight. If you are at a healthy weight, aim to avoid weight gain. If you are already overweight, first aim to prevent further weight gain, and then lose weight to improve your health.

Build a healthy base by eating vegetables, fruits, and grains (especially whole grains) with little added fat or sugar.

Select sensible portion sizes.

Get moving. Get regular physical activity to balance calories from the foods you eat.

Set a good example for children by practicing healthy eating habits and enjoying regular physical activities together.

Keep in mind that even though heredity and the environment are important influences, your behaviors help determine your body weight.

Be Physically active each day

Being physically active and maintaining a healthy weight are both needed for good health, but they benefit health in different ways. Children, teens, adults, and the elderly—all can improve their health and well-being and have fun by including moderate amounts of physical activity in their daily lives. Physical activity involves moving the body. A moderate physical activity is any activity that requires about as much energy as walking 2 miles in 30 minutes.

Aim to accumulate at least 30 minutes (adults) or 60 minutes (children) of moderate physical activity most days of the week, preferably daily. If you already get 30 minutes of physical activity daily, you can gain even more health benefits by increasing the amount of time that you are physically active or by taking part in more vigorous activities. No matter what activity you choose, you can do it all at once, or spread it out over two or three times during the day.

Make physical activity a regular part of your routine

Choose activities that you enjoy and that you can do regularly (see INDEX 4). Some people prefer activities that fit into their daily routine, like gardening or taking extra trips up and down stairs. Others prefer a regular exercise program, such as a physical activity program at their worksite. Some do both. The important thing is to be physically active every day.

Most adults do not need to see their health care provider before starting to become more physically active. However, if you are planning to start a vigorous activity plan and have one or more of the conditions below, consult your health care provider:

Chronic health problem such as heart disease, hypertension, diabetes, osteoporosis, or obesity.

High risk for heart disease (see INDEX 2).

Over age 40 for men or 50 for women.

Health benefits of physical activity

Compared with being very sedentary, being physically active for at least 30 minutes on most days of the week reduces the risk of developing or dying of heart disease. It has other health benefits as well (see INDEX 5). No one is too young or too old to enjoy the benefits of regular physical activity.

Two types of physical activity are especially beneficial:

Aerobic activities. These are activities that speed your heart rate and breathing. They help cardiovascular fitness.

Activities for strength and flexibility. Developing strength may help build and maintain your bones. Carrying groceries and lifting weights are two strength-building activities. Gentle stretching, dancing, or yoga can increase flexibility.

To get these health benefits, adults need moderate physical activity for a total of at least 30 minutes most days of the week, preferably daily, and children need at least 60 minutes per day.

INDEX 4

EXAMPLES OF PHYSICAL ACTIVITIES FOR ADULTS

For at least 30 minutes most days of the week, preferably daily, do any one of the activities listed below—or combine activities. Look for additional opportunities among other activities that you enjoy.

As part of your routine activities:

- Walk, wheel, or bike ride more, drive less.
- Walk up stairs instead of taking an elevator.
- Get off the bus a few stops early and walk or wheel the remaining distance.
- Mow the lawn with a push mower.
- Rake leaves.
- Garden.
- Push a stroller.
- Clean the house.
- Do exercises or pedal a stationary bike while watching television.
- Play actively with children.
- Take a brisk 10-minute walk or wheel in the morning, at lunch, and after dinner.

As part of your exercise or recreational routine:

- Walk, wheel, or jog.
- Bicycle or use an arm pedal bicycle.
- Swim or do water aerobics.
- Play racket or wheelchair sports.

- Golf (pull cart or carry clubs).
- Canoe.
- Cross-country ski.
- Play basketball.
- Dance.
- Take part in an exercise program at work, home, school, or gym.

INDEX 5

HEALTH BENEFITS OF REGULAR PHYSICAL ACTIVITY

- Increases physical fitness.
- Helps build and maintain healthy bones, muscles, and joints.
- Builds endurance and muscular strength.
- Helps manage weight.
- Lowers risk factors for cardiovascular disease, colon cancer, and type 2 diabetes.
- Helps control blood pressure.
- Promotes psychological well-being and self-esteem.
- Reduces feelings of depression and anxiety.

Physical activity and nutrition

Physical activity and nutrition work together for better health. For example, physical activity increases the amount of calories you use. For those who have intentionally lost weight, being active makes it easier to maintain the weight loss. However, 30 minutes of activity daily may not be enough to lose weight or maintain weight loss. Read the preceding guideline "Aim for a Healthy Weight," for more information about weight management.

Physical activity and nutrition work together in more ways than weight management. Increasing the calories you use allows you to eat more, which makes it easier to get the nutrients you need. Physical activity and nutrition work together for bone health, too. Calcium and other nutrients are needed to build and maintain strong bones, but physical activity is needed as well.

Help children be physically active

Children and adolescents benefit from physical activity in many ways. They need at least 60 minutes of physical activity daily (see INDEX 6). Parents can help:

Set a good example. For example, arrange active family events in which everyone takes part. Join your children in physical activities.

Encourage your children to be physically active at home, at school, and with friends by jumping rope, playing tag, riding a bike.

Limit television watching, computer games, and other inactive forms of play by alternating with periods of physical activity.

INDEX 6

PHYSICAL ACTIVITIES FOR CHILDREN AND TEENS

Aim for at least 60 minutes total per day:

- Be spontaneously active.
- Play tag.
- Jump rope.
- Ride a bicycle or tricycle.
- Walk, wheel, skip, or run.
- Play actively during school recess.
- Roller skate or in-line skate.
- Take part in physical education activity classes during school.
- Join after-school or community physical activity programs.
- Dance.

Older people need to be physically active too

Older persons also need to be physically active. Engage in moderate physical activity for at least 30 minutes most days of the week, preferably daily, and taking part in activities to strengthen muscles and to improve flexibility. Staying strong and flexible can reduce your risk of falling and breaking bones, preserve muscle, and improve your ability to live independently. Lifting small weights and carrying groceries are two ways to include strength building into your routine.

Engage in at least 30 minutes (adults) or 60 minutes (children) of moderate physical activity most, preferably all, days of the week.

Become physically active if you are inactive.

Maintain or increase physical activity if you are already active.

Stay active throughout your life.

Help children get at least 60 minutes of physical activity daily.

Choose physical activities that fit in with your daily routine, or choose recreational or structured exercise programs, or both.

Consult your health care provider before starting a new vigorous physical activity plan if you have a chronic health problem, or if you are over 40 (men) or 50 (women).

Different foods contain different nutrients and other healthful substances. No single food can supply all the nutrients in the amounts you need. For example, oranges provide vitamin C and folate but no vitamin B12; cheese provides calcium and vitamin B12; but no vitamin C. To make sure you get all the nutrients and other substances you need for health, build a healthy base by using the Food Guide Pyramid as a starting point. Choose the recommended number of daily servings from each of the five major food groups (INDEX 7). If you avoid all foods from any of the five food groups, seek guidance to help ensure that you get all the nutrients you need.

INDEX 7

HOW MANY SERVINGS DO YOU NEED EACH DAY?

Food group Children ages 2 to 6 years, women, some older adults (about 1,600 calories) Older children, teen girls, active women, most men (about 2,200 calories)

Teen boys, active men (about 2,800 calories)

Bread, Cereal, Rice, and Pasta Group (Grains Group)—especially whole grain6 9 11
Vegetable Group 3 4 5
Fruit Group 2 3 4
Milk, Yogurt, and Cheese Group (Milk Group)—preferably fat free or low fat 2 or 3* 2 or 3* 2 or 3*

Meat, Poultry, Fish, Dry Beans, Eggs, and Nuts Group (Meat and Beans Group)—preferably lean or low fat2, for a total of 5 ounces 2, for a total of 6 ounces 3, for a total of 7 ounces
Adapted from U.S. Department of Agriculture, Center for Nutrition Policy and Promotion. The Food Guide Pyramid, Home and Garden Bulletin Number 252, 1996. *

The number of servings depends on your age. Older children and teenagers (ages 9 to 18 years) and adults over the age of 50 need 3 servings daily. Others need 2 servings daily. During pregnancy and lactation, the recommended number of milk group servings is the same as for nonpregnant women.

Figure 2

INDEX 8

WHAT COUNTS AS A SERVING?

Bread, Cereal, Rice, and Pasta Group (Grains Group)—whole grain and refined

- 1 slice of bread
- About 1 cup of ready-to-eat cereal
- ½ cup of cooked cereal, rice, or pasta

Vegetable Group

- 1 cup of raw leafy vegetables
- ½ cup of other vegetables cooked or raw
- ¾ cup of vegetable juice

Fruit Group

- 1 medium apple, banana, orange, pear

- ½ cup of chopped, cooked, or canned fruit
- ¾ cup of fruit juice

Milk, Yogurt, and Cheese Group (Milk Group)*

- 1 cup of milk** or yogurt**
- 1 ½ ounces of natural cheese** (such as Cheddar)
- 2 ounces of processed cheese** (such as American)

Meat, Poultry, Fish, Dry Beans, Eggs, and Nuts Group (Meat and Beans Group)

- 2-3 ounces of cooked lean meat, poultry, or fish
- ½ cup of cooked dry beans# or ½ cup of tofu counts as 1 ounce of lean meat
- 2 ½-ounce soyburger or 1 egg counts as 1 ounce of lean meat
- 2 tablespoons of peanut butter or 1/3 cup of nuts counts as 1 ounce of meat

NOTE: Many of the serving sizes given above are smaller than those on the Nutrition Facts Label. For example, 1 serving of cooked cereal, rice, or pasta is 1 cup for the label but only ½ cup for the Pyramid.

- This includes lactose-free and lactose-reduced milk products. One cup of soy-based beverage with added calcium is an option for those who prefer a non-dairy source of calcium.
- Choose fat-free or reduced-fat dairy products most often.

Dry beans, peas, and lentils can be counted as servings in either the meat and beans group or the vegetable group. As a vegetable, ½ cup of cooked, dry beans counts as 1 serving. As a meat substitute, 1 cup of cooked, dry beans counts as 1 serving (2 ounces of meat).

Use plant foods as the foundation of your meals

There are many ways to create a healthy eating pattern, but they all start with the three food groups at the base of the Pyramid: grains, fruits, and vegetables. Eating a variety of grains (especially whole grain foods), fruits, and vegetables is the basis of healthy eating. Enjoy meals that have rice, pasta, tortillas, or whole grain bread at the center of the plate, accompanied by plenty of fruits and vegetables and a moderate amount of low-fat foods from the milk group and the meat and beans group. Go easy on foods high in fat or sugars.

Keep an eye on servings

Compare the recommended number of servings in INDEX 7 and the serving sizes in INDEX 8 with what you usually eat. If you don't need many calories (because you're inactive, for example), aim for the lower number of servings. Notice that some of the serving sizes in INDEX 8 are smaller than what you might usually eat or see on food labels. For example, many people eat 2 slices of bread in a meal, which equal 2 servings. So it's easy to meet the recommended number of servings. Young children 2 to 3 years old need the same number of servings as others, but smaller serving sizes except for milk.

Also, notice that many of the meals and snacks you eat contain items from several food groups. For example, a sandwich may provide bread from the grains group, turkey from the meat and beans group, and cheese from the milk group.

Choose a variety of foods for good nutrition. Since foods within most food groups differ in their content of nutrients and other beneficial substances, choosing a variety helps you get all the nutrients and fiber you need. It can also help keep your meals interesting from day to day.

There are many healthful eating patterns

Different people like different foods and like to prepare the same foods in different ways. Culture, family background, religion, moral beliefs, the cost and availability of food, life experiences, food intolerances, and allergies affect people's food choices. Use the Food Guide Pyramid as a starting point to shape your eating pattern. It provides a good guide to make sure you get enough nutrients. Make choices from each major group in the Food Guide Pyramid, and combine them however you like. For example, those who like Mexican cuisine might choose tortillas from the grains group and beans from the meat and beans group, while those who eat Asian food might choose rice from the grains group and tofu from the meat and beans group.

If you usually avoid all foods from one or two of the food groups, be sure to get enough nutrients from other food groups. For example, if you choose not to eat milk products because of intolerance to lactose or for other reasons, choose other foods that are good sources of calcium (see INDEX 9), and be sure to get enough vitamin D. Meat, fish, and poultry are major contributors of iron, zinc, and B vitamins in most American diets. If you choose to avoid all or most animal products, be sure to get enough iron, vitamin B12, calcium, and zinc from other sources. Vegetarian diets can be consistent with the Dietary Guidelines for Americans, and meet Recommended Dietary Allowances for nutrients.

INDEX 9

SOME SOURCES OF CALCIUM*

- Yogurt#
- Milk**#
- Natural cheeses such as Mozzarella, Cheddar, Swiss, and Parmesan#
- Soy-based beverage with added calcium
- Tofu, if made with calcium sulfate (read the ingredient list)
- Breakfast cereal with added calcium
- Canned fish with soft bones such as salmon, sardines†
- Fruit juice with added calcium
- Pudding made with milk#
- Soup made with milk#
- Dark-green leafy vegetables such as collards, turnip greens

• Read food labels for brand-specific information

** This includes lactose-free and lactose-reduced milk.

Choose low-fat or fat-free milk products most often.

† High in salt.

Growing children, teenagers, women, and older adults have higher needs for some nutrients

Adolescents and adults over age 50 have an especially high need for calcium, but most people need to eat plenty of good sources of calcium for healthy bones throughout life. When selecting dairy products to get enough calcium, choose those that are low in fat or fat-free to avoid getting too much saturated fat. Young children, teenage girls, and women of childbearing age need enough good sources of iron, such as lean meats and cereals with added nutrients, to keep up their iron stores (see INDEX 10). Women who could become pregnant need extra folic acid, and older adults need extra vitamin D.

INDEX 10

SOME SOURCES OF IRON*

- Shellfish like shrimp, clams, mussels, and oysters
- Lean meats (especially beef), liver** and other organ meats**
- Ready-to-eat cereals with added iron
- Turkey dark meat (remove skin to reduce fat)
- Sardines†
- Spinach
- Cooked dry beans (such as kidney beans and pinto beans), peas (such as black-eyed peas), and lentils
- Enriched and whole grain breads

- Read food labels for brand-specific information.

** Very high in cholesterol.

† High in salt.

Check the food label before you buy

Food labels have several parts, including the front panel, Nutrition Facts, and ingredient list. The front panel often tells you if nutrients have been added—for example, "iodized salt" lets you know that iodine has been added, and "enriched pasta" (or "enriched" grain of any type) means that thiamin, riboflavin, niacin, iron, and folic acid have been added.

The ingredient list tells you what's in the food, including any nutrients, fats, or sugars that have been added. The ingredients are listed in descending order by weight.

Use the Nutrition Facts to see if a food is a good source of a nutrient or to compare similar foods—for example, to find which brand of frozen dinner is lower in saturated fat, or which kind of breakfast cereal contains more folic acid. Look at the % Daily Value (%DV) column to see whether a food is high or low in nutrients. If you want to limit a nutrient (such as fat, saturated fat, cholesterol, sodium), try to choose foods with a lower %DV. If you want to consume more of a nutrient (such as calcium, other vitamins and minerals, fiber), try to choose foods with a higher %DV. As a guide, foods with 5%DV or less contribute a small amount of that nutrient to your eating pattern, while those with 20% or more contribute a large amount. Remember, Nutrition Facts serving sizes may differ from those used in the Food Guide Pyramid (see INDEX 8). For example, 2 ounces of dry macaroni yields about 1 cup cooked, or two (1/2 cup) Pyramid servings.

Use of dietary supplements

Some people need a vitamin-mineral supplement to meet specific nutrient needs. For example, women who could become pregnant are advised to eat foods fortified with folic acid or to take a folic acid supplement in addition to consuming folate-rich foods to reduce the risk of some serious birth defects. Older adults and people with little exposure to sunlight may need a vitamin D supplement. People who seldom eat dairy products or other rich sources of calcium need a calcium supplement, and people who eat no animal foods need to take a vitamin B12 supplement. Sometimes vitamins or minerals are prescribed for meeting nutrient needs or for therapeutic purposes. For example, health care providers may advise pregnant women to take an iron supplement, and adults over age 50 to get their vitamin B12 from a supplement or from fortified foods.

Supplements of some nutrients, such as vitamin A and selenium, can be harmful if taken in large amounts. Because foods contain many substances that promote health, use the Food Guide Pyramid when choosing foods.

Don't depend on supplements to meet your usual nutrient needs.

Dietary supplements include not only vitamins and minerals, but also amino acids, fiber, herbal products, and many other substances that are widely available. Herbal products usually provide a very small amount of vitamins and minerals. The value of herbal products for health is currently being studied. Standards for their purity, potency, and composition are being developed.

Build a healthy base: Use the Food Guide Pyramid to help make healthy food choices that you can enjoy.

Build your eating pattern on a variety of plant foods, including whole grains, fruits, and vegetables.

Also choose some low-fat dairy products and low-fat foods from the meat and beans group each day.

It's fine to enjoy fats and sweets occasionally.

Choose a variety of grains daily, especially whole grains

Foods made from grains (wheat, rice, and oats) help form the foundation of a nutritious diet. They provide vitamins, minerals, carbohydrates (starch and dietary fiber), and other substances that are important for good health. Grain products are low in fat, unless fat is added in processing, in preparation, or at the table. Whole grains differ from refined grains in the amount of fiber and nutrients they provide, and different whole grain foods differ in nutrient content, so choose a variety of whole and enriched grains. Eating plenty of whole grains, such as whole wheat bread or oatmeal (see INDEX 11), as part of the healthful eating patterns described by these guidelines, may help protect you against many chronic diseases. Aim for at least 6 servings of grain products per day—more if you are an older child or teenager, an adult man, or an active woman (see INDEX 7)—and include several servings of whole grain foods. See INDEX 8 for serving sizes.

Why choose whole grain foods?

Vitamins, minerals, fiber, and other protective substances in whole grain foods contribute to the health benefits of whole grains. Refined grains are low in fiber and in the protective substances that accompany fiber. Eating plenty of fiber-containing foods, such as whole grains (and also many fruits and vegetables) promotes proper bowel function. The high fiber content of many whole grains may also help you to feel full with fewer calories. Fiber is best obtained from foods like whole grains, fruits, and vegetables rather than from fiber supplements for several reasons: there are many types of fiber, the composition of fiber is poorly understood, and other protective substances accompany fiber in foods. Use the Nutrition Facts Label to help choose grains that are rich in fiber and low in saturated fat and sodium.

INDEX 11

HOW TO INCREASE YOUR INTAKE OF WHOLE GRAIN FOODS

Choose foods that name one of the following ingredients first on the label's ingredient list (see sample in figure 4).

- brown rice
- oatmeal
- whole oats
- bulgur (cracked wheat)
- popcorn
- whole rye
- graham flour
- pearl barley
- whole wheat
- whole grain corn

Try some of these whole grain foods: whole wheat bread, whole grain ready-to-eat cereal, low-fat whole wheat crackers, oatmeal, whole wheat pasta, whole barley in soup, tabouli salad.

NOTE: "Wheat flour," "enriched flour," and "degerminated corn meal" are not whole grains.

SAMPLE INGREDIENT LIST FOR A WHOLE GRAIN FOOD

INGREDIENTS: WHOLE WHEAT FLOUR, WATER, HIGH FRUCTOSE CORN SYRUP, WHEAT GLUTEN, SOYBEAN AND/ OR CANOLA OIL, YEAST, SALT, HONEY.

Enriched grains are a new source of folic acid

Folic acid, a form of folate, is now added to all enriched grain products (thiamin, riboflavin, niacin, and iron have been added to enriched grains for many years). Folate is a B vitamin that reduces the risk of some serious types of birth defects when consumed before and during early pregnancy. Studies are underway to clarify whether it decreases risk for coronary heart disease, stroke, and certain types of cancer. Whole grain foods naturally contain some folate, but only a few (mainly ready-to-eat breakfast cereals) contain added folic acid as well. Read the ingredient label to find out if folic acid and other nutrients have been added, and check the Nutrition Facts Label to compare the nutrient content of foods like breakfast cereals.

Build a healthy base by making a variety of grain products a foundation of your diet.

Eat 6 or more servings of grain products daily (whole grain and refined breads, cereals, pasta, and rice). Include several servings of whole grain foods daily for their good taste and their health benefits. If your calorie needs are low, have only 6 servings of a sensible size daily (see INDEX 8 for examples of serving sizes).

Eat foods made from a variety of whole grains—such as whole wheat, brown rice, oats, and whole grain corn—every day.

Combine whole grains with other tasty, nutritious foods in mixed dishes.

Prepare or choose grain products with little added saturated fat and a moderate or low amount of added sugars. Also, check the sodium content on the Nutrition Facts Label.

Choose a variety of fruits and vegetables daily

Fruits and vegetables are key parts of your daily diet. Eating plenty of fruits and vegetables of different kinds, as part of the healthful eating patterns described by these guidelines, may help protect you against many chronic diseases. It also promotes healthy bowel function. Fruits and vegetables provide essential vitamins and minerals, fiber, and other substances that are important for good health. Most people, including children, eat fewer servings of fruits and vegetables than are recommended. To promote your health, eat a variety of fruits and vegetables—at least 2 servings of fruits and 3 servings of vegetables—each day.

Why eat plenty of different fruits and vegetables?

Different fruits and vegetables are rich in different nutrients (see INDEX 12). Some fruits and vegetables are excellent sources of carotenoids, including those which form vitamin A, while others may be rich in vitamin C, folate, or potassium. Fruits and vegetables, especially dry beans and peas, also contain fiber and other substances that are associated with good health. Dark-green leafy vegetables, deeply colored fruits, and dry beans and peas are especially rich in many nutrients. Most fruits and vegetables are naturally low in fat and calories and are filling. Some are high in fiber, and many are quick to prepare and easy to eat. Choose whole or cut-up fruits and vegetables rather than juices most often. Juices contain little or no fiber.

INDEX 12

WHICH FRUITS AND VEGETABLES PROVIDE THE MOST NUTRIENTS?

The lists below show which fruits and vegetables are the best sources of vitamin A (carotenoids), vitamin C, folate, and potassium. Eat at least 2 servings of fruits and at least 3 servings of vegetables each day:

Sources of vitamin A (carotenoids)

- Orange vegetables like carrots, sweet potatoes, pumpkin
- Dark-green leafy vegetables such as spinach, collards, turnip greens
- Orange fruits like mango, cantaloupe, apricots
- Tomatoes

Sources of vitamin C

- Citrus fruits and juices, kiwi fruit, strawberries, cantaloupe
- Broccoli, peppers, tomatoes, cabbage, potatoes
- Leafy greens such as romaine lettuce, turnip greens, spinach

Sources of folate

- Cooked dry beans and peas, peanuts
- Oranges, orange juice
- Dark-green leafy vegetables like spinach and mustard greens, romaine lettuce
- Green peas

Sources of potassium

- Baked white or sweet potato, cooked greens (such as spinach), winter (orange) squash
- Bananas, plantains, dried fruits such as apricots and prunes, orange juice
- Cooked dry beans (such as baked beans) and lentils

NOTE: Read Nutrition Facts Labels for product-specific information, especially for processed fruits and vegetables.

Aim for Variety

Try many colors and kinds. Choose any form: fresh, frozen, canned, dried, juices. All forms provide vitamins and minerals, and all provide fiber except for most juices—so choose fruits and vegetables most often. Wash fresh fruits and vegetables thoroughly before using. If you buy prepared vegetables, check the Nutrition Facts Label to find choices that are low in saturated fat and sodium.

Try serving fruits and vegetables in new ways:

raw vegetables with a low- or reduced-fat dip

vegetables stir-fried in a small amount of vegetable oil

fruits or vegetables mixed with other foods in salads, casseroles, soups, sauces (for example, add shredded vegetables when making meatloaf)

Find ways to include plenty of different fruits and vegetables in your meals and snacks.

Buy wisely. Frozen or canned fruits and vegetables are sometimes best buys, and they are rich in nutrients. If fresh fruit is very ripe, buy only enough to use right away.

Store properly to maintain quality. Refrigerate most fresh fruits (not bananas) and vegetables (not potatoes or tomatoes) for longer storage, and arrange them so you'll use up the ripest ones first. If you cut them up or open a can, cover and refrigerate afterward.

Keep ready-to-eat raw vegetables handy in a clear container in the front of your refrigerator for snacks or meals-on-the-go.

Keep a day's supply of fresh or dried fruit handy on the table or counter.

Enjoy fruits as a naturally sweet end to a meal.

When eating out, choose a variety of vegetables at a salad bar.

Enjoy 5 a day—eat at least 2 servings of fruit and at least 3 servings of vegetables each day (see INDEX 8 for serving sizes).

Choose fresh, frozen, dried, or canned forms and a variety of colors and kinds.

Choose dark-green leafy vegetables, orange fruits and vegetables, and cooked dry beans and peas often.

Keep food safe to eat

Foods that are safe from harmful bacteria, viruses, parasites, and chemical contaminants are vital for healthful eating. Safe means that the food poses little risk of foodborne illness (see INDEX 13). Farmers, food producers, markets, food service establishments, and other food preparers have a role to keep food as safe as possible. However, we also need to keep and prepare foods safely in the home, and be alert when eating out.

INDEX 13

WHAT IS FOODBORNE ILLNESS?

Foodborne illness is caused by eating food that contains harmful bacteria, toxins, parasites, viruses, or chemical contaminants. Bacteria and viruses, especially Campylobacter, Salmonella, and Norwalk-like viruses, are among the most common causes of foodborne illness we know about today. Eating even a small portion of an unsafe food may make you sick. Signs and symptoms may appear within half an hour of eating a contaminated food or may not develop for up to 3 weeks. Most foodborne illness lasts a few hours or days. Some foodborne illnesses have effects that go on for weeks, months, or even years. If you think you have become ill from eating a food, consult your health care provider.

Follow the steps below to keep your food safe. Be very careful with perishable foods such as eggs, meats, poultry, fish, shellfish, milk products, and fresh fruits and vegetables. If you are at high risk of foodborne illness, be extra careful (see INDEX 14).

INDEX 14

TIPS FOR THOSE AT HIGH RISK OF FOODBORNE ILLNESS

Who is at high risk of foodborne illness?

- Pregnant women
- Young children
- Older persons
- People with weakened immune systems or certain chronic illnesses

Besides following the guidance in this guideline, some of the extra precautions those at high risk should take are:

- Do not eat or drink unpasteurized juices, raw sprouts, raw (unpasteurized) milk and products made from unpasteurized milk.

- Do not eat raw or undercooked meat, poultry, eggs, fish, and shellfish (clams, oysters, scallops, and mussels).

New information on food safety is constantly emerging. Recommendations and precautions for people at high risk are updated as scientists learn more about preventing foodborne illness. If you are among those at high risk, you need to be aware of and follow the most current information on food safety.

Clean. Wash hands and surfaces often

Wash your hands with warm soapy water for 20 seconds (count to 30) before you handle food or food utensils. Wash your hands after handling or preparing food, especially after handling raw meat, poultry, fish, shellfish, or eggs. Right after you prepare these raw foods, clean the utensils and surfaces you used with hot soapy water. Replace cutting boards once they have become worn or develop hard-to-clean grooves. Wash raw fruit and vegetables under running water before eating. Use a vegetable brush to remove surface dirt if necessary. Always wash your hands after using the bathroom, changing diapers, or playing with pets. When eating out, if the tables, dinnerware, and restrooms look dirty, the kitchen may be, too—so you may want to eat somewhere else.

Separate raw, cooked, and ready-to-eat foods while shopping, preparing, or storing

Keep raw meat, poultry, eggs, fish, and shellfish away from other foods, surfaces, utensils, or serving plates. This prevents cross-contamination from one food to another. Store raw meat, poultry, fish, and shellfish in containers in the refrigerator so that the juices don't drip onto other foods.

Cook. Cook foods to a safe temperature

Uncooked and undercooked animal foods are potentially unsafe. Proper cooking makes most uncooked foods safe. The best way to tell if meat, poultry, or egg dishes are cooked to a safe temperature is to use a food thermometer (figure 5). Several kinds of inexpensive food thermometers are available in many stores.

Reheat sauces, soups, marinades, and gravies to a boil. Reheat leftovers thoroughly to at least 165° F. If using a microwave oven, cover the container and turn or stir the food to make sure it is heated evenly throughout. Cook eggs until whites and yolks are firm. Don't eat raw or partially cooked eggs, or foods containing raw eggs, raw (unpasteurized) milk, or cheeses made with raw milk. Choose pasteurized juices. The risk of contamination is high from undercooked hamburger, and from raw fish (including sushi), clams, and oysters. Cook fish and shellfish until it is opaque; fish should flake easily with a fork. When eating out, order foods thoroughly cooked and make sure they are served piping hot.

Chill. Refrigerate perishable foods promptly

When shopping, buy perishable foods last, and take them straight home. At home, refrigerate or freeze meat, poultry, eggs, fish, shellfish, ready-to-eat foods, and leftovers promptly. Refrigerate within 2 hours of purchasing or preparation—and within 1 hour if the air temperature is above 90° F. Refrigerate at or below 40° F, or freeze at or below 0° F. Use refrigerated leftovers within 3 to 4 days. Freeze fresh meat, poultry, fish, and shellfish that cannot be used in a few days. Thaw frozen meat, poultry, fish, and shellfish in the refrigerator, microwave, or cold water changed every 30 minutes. (This keeps the surface chilled.) Cook foods immediately after thawing. Never thaw meat, poultry, fish, or shellfish at room temperature. When eating out, make sure that any foods you order that should be refrigerated are served chilled.

Follow the label

Read the label and follow safety instructions on the package such as "KEEP REFRIGERATED" and the "SAFE HANDLING INSTRUCTIONS."

Serve safely

Keep hot foods hot (140° F or above) and cold foods cold (40° F or below). Harmful bacteria can grow rapidly in the "danger zone" between these temperatures. Whether raw or cooked, never leave meat, poultry, eggs, fish, or shellfish out at room temperature for more than 2 hours (1 hour in hot weather 90° F or above). Be sure to chill leftovers as soon as you are finished eating. These guidelines also apply to carry-out meals, restaurant leftovers, and home-packed meals-to-go.

When in doubt, throw it out

If you aren't sure that food has been prepared, served, or stored safely, throw it out. You may not be able to make food safe if it has been handled in an unsafe manner. For example, a food that has been left at room temperature too long may contain a toxin produced by bacteria—one that can't be destroyed by cooking. So if meat, poultry, fish, shellfish, or eggs have been left out for more than 2 hours, or if the food has been kept in the refrigerator too long, don't taste it. Just throw it out. Even if it looks and smells fine, it may not be safe to eat. If you have doubt when you're shopping or eating out, choose something else. For more information, contact USDA's Meat and Poultry Hotline, 1-800-535-4555, or FDA's Food Information Line, 1-888-SAFE FOOD. Also, ask your local or state health department or Cooperative Extension Service Office for further guidance.

Build a healthy base by keeping food safe to eat.

Clean. Wash hands and surfaces often.

Separate. Separate raw, cooked, and ready-to-eat foods while shopping, preparing, or storing.

Cook. Cook foods to a safe temperature.
Chill. Refrigerate perishable foods promptly.
Check and follow the label.
Serve safely. Keep hot foods hot and cold foods cold.
When in doubt, throw it out.

Choose a diet that is low in saturated fat and cholesterol and moderate in total fat

Fats supply energy and essential fatty acids, and they help absorb the fat-soluble vitamins A, D, E, and K, and carotenoids. You need some fat in the food you eat, but choose sensibly. Some kinds of fat, especially saturated fats, increase the risk for coronary heart disease by raising the blood cholesterol (see INDEX 15). In contrast, unsaturated fats (found mainly in vegetable oils) do not increase blood cholesterol. Fat intake in the United States as a proportion of total calories is lower than it was many years ago, but most people still eat too much saturated fat. Eating lots of fat of any type can provide excess calories.

Choose foods low in saturated fat and cholesterol

See INDEX 16 for tips on limiting the amount of saturated fat and cholesterol you get from your food. Taking these steps can go a long way in helping to keep your blood cholesterol level low.

INDEX 15

KNOW THE DIFFERENT TYPES OF FATS

Saturated Fats

Foods high in saturated fats tend to raise blood cholesterol. These foods include high-fat dairy products (like cheese, whole milk, cream, butter, and regular ice cream), fatty fresh and processed meats, the skin and fat of poultry, lard, palm oil, and coconut oil. Keep your intake of these foods low.

Dietary Cholesterol

Foods that are high in cholesterol also tend to raise blood cholesterol. These foods include liver and other organ meats, egg yolks, and dairy fats.

Trans Fatty Acids

Foods high in trans fatty acids tend to raise blood cholesterol. These foods include those high in partially hydrogenated vegetable oils, such as many hard margarines and shortenings. Foods with a high amount of these ingredients include some commercially fried foods and some bakery goods.

Unsaturated Fats

Unsaturated fats (oils) do not raise blood cholesterol. Unsaturated fats occur in vegetable oils, most nuts, olives, avocados, and fatty fish like salmon. Unsaturated oils include both monounsaturated fats and polyunsaturated fats. Olive, canola, sunflower, and peanut oils are some of the oils high in monounsaturated fats. Vegetable oils such as soybean oil, corn oil, and cottonseed oil and many kinds of nuts are good sources of polyunsaturated fats. Some fish, such as salmon, tuna, and mackerel, contain omega-3 fatty acids that are being studied to determine if they offer protection against heart disease. Use moderate amounts of food high in unsaturated fats, taking care to avoid excess calories.

INDEX 16

FOOD CHOICES LOW IN SATURATED FAT AND CHOLESTEROL AND MODERATE IN TOTAL FAT

Get most of your calories from plant foods (grains, fruits, vegetables). If you eat foods high in saturated fat for a special occasion, return to foods that are low in saturated fat the next day.

Fats and Oils

- Choose vegetable oils rather than solid fats (meat and dairy fats, shortening).
- If you need fewer calories, decrease the amount of fat you use in cooking and at the table.

Meat, Poultry, Fish, Shellfish, Eggs, Beans, and Nuts

- Choose 2 to 3 servings of fish, shellfish, lean poultry, other lean meats, beans, or nuts daily. Trim fat from meat and take skin off poultry. Choose dry beans, peas, or lentils often.
- Limit your intake of high-fat processed meats such as bacon, sausages, salami, bologna, and other cold cuts. Try the lower fat varieties (check the Nutrition Facts Label).
- Limit your intake of liver and other organ meats. Use egg yolks and whole eggs in moderation. Use egg whites

and egg substitutes freely when cooking since they contain no cholesterol and little or no fat.

Dairy Products

- Choose fat-free or low-fat milk, fat-free or low-fat yogurt, and low-fat cheese most often. Try switching from whole to fat-free or low-fat milk. This decreases the saturated fat and calories but keeps all other nutrients the same.

Prepared Foods

- Check the Nutrition Facts Label to see how much saturated fat and cholesterol are in a serving of prepared food. Choose foods lower in saturated fat and cholesterol.

Foods at Restaurants or Other Eating Establishments

- Choose fish or lean meats as suggested above. Limit ground meat and fatty processed meats, marbled steaks, and cheese.
- Limit your intake of foods with creamy sauces, and add little or no butter to your food.
- Choose fruits as desserts most often.

Following the tips in the INDEX above will help you keep your intake of saturated fat at less than 10 percent of calories. They will also help you keep your cholesterol intake less than the Daily Value of 300 mg/day listed on the Nutrition Facts Label. If you want more flexibility, see INDEX 17, below, to find out your saturated fat limit in grams. The maximum number of saturated fat grams depends on the amount of calories you get daily. Use Nutrition Facts Labels to find out how much saturated fat is in prepared foods. If you choose one food that is higher in saturated fat, make your other choices lower in saturated fat. This will help you stay under your saturated fat limit for the day.

INDEX 17

WHAT IS YOUR UPPER LIMIT ON FAT FOR THE CALORIES YOU CONSUME?

Total Calories per Day	Saturated Fat in Grams	Total Fat in Grams
1,600	18 or less	53
2,000*	20 or less	65
2,200	24 or less	73
2,500*	25 or less	80
2,800	31 or less	93

- Percent Daily Values on Nutrition Facts Labels are based on a 2,000 calorie diet. Values for 2,000 and 2,500 calories are rounded to the nearest 5 grams to be consistent with the Nutrition Facts Label.

Different forms of the same food may be very different in their content of saturated fat. INDEX 18 provides some examples. Try to choose the forms of food that are lower in saturated fat most often.

Keep total fat intake moderate

Aim for a total fat intake of no more than 30 percent of calories, as recommended in previous editions of the Guidelines. If you need to reduce your fat intake to achieve this level, do so primarily by cutting back on saturated and trans fats. Check INDEX 17 to find out how many grams of fat you can have for the number of calories you need. For example, at 2,200 calories per day, your suggested upper limit on fat intake would be about 73 grams. If you are at a healthy weight and you eat little saturated fat, you'll have leeway to eat some plant foods that are high in unsaturated fats. To see if you need to lose weight, see the guideline "Aim for a Healthy Weight."

Advice for children

Advice in the previous sections applies to children who are 2 years of age or older. It does not apply to infants and toddlers below the age of 2 years. Beginning at age 2, children should get most of their calories from grain products; fruits; vegetables; low-fat dairy products; and beans, lean meat and poultry, fish, or nuts. Be careful, nuts may cause choking in 2 to 3 year olds.

To reduce your intake of saturated fat and cholesterol:

Limit use of solid fats, such as butter, hard margarines, lard, and partially hydrogenated shortenings. Use vegetable oils as a substitute.

Choose fat-free or low-fat dairy products, cooked dry beans and peas, fish, and lean meats and poultry.

Eat plenty of grain products, vegetables, and fruits daily.

Use the Nutrition Facts Label to help choose foods lower in fat, saturated fat, and cholesterol.

INDEX 18

A COMPARISON OF SATURATED FAT IN SOME FOODS

Food Category	Portion	Saturated Fat Content in Grams
Cheese		
Regular Cheddar cheese	1 oz	6.0
Low-fat Cheddar cheese*	1 oz.	1.2
Ground Beef		
Regular ground beef	3 oz. cooked	7.2
Extra lean ground beef*	3 oz. cooked	5.3
Milk		
Whole milk	1 cup	5.1
Low-fat (1%) milk*	1 cup	1.6
Breads		
Croissant	1 medium	6.6
Bagel*	1 medium	0.1
Frozen Desserts		
Regular ice cream	1/2 cup	4.5
Frozen yogurt*	1/2 cup	2.5
Table Spreads		
Butter	1 tsp.	2.4
Soft margarine*	1 tsp.	0.7

NOTE: The food categories listed are among the major food sources of saturated fat for U.S. adults and children.

*** Choice that is lower in saturated fat.**

Choose beverages and foods to moderate your intake of sugars

Sugars are carbohydrates and a source of energy (calories). Dietary carbohydrates also include the complex carbohydrates starch and dietary fiber. During digestion all carbohydrates except fiber break down into sugars. Sugars and starches occur naturally in many foods that also supply other nutrients. Examples of these foods include milk, fruits, some vegetables, breads, cereals, and grains.

Sugars and tooth decay

Foods containing sugars and starches can promote tooth decay. The amount of bacteria in your mouth and lack of exposure to fluorides also promote tooth decay. These bacteria use sugars and starches to produce the acid that causes tooth decay.

The more often you eat foods that contain sugars and starches, and the longer these foods remain in your mouth before you brush your teeth, the greater your risk for tooth decay. Frequent eating or drinking sweet or starchy foods between meals is more likely to harm teeth than eating the same foods at meals and then brushing. Daily dental hygiene, including brushing with fluoride toothpaste and flossing, and adequate intake of fluorides will help prevent tooth decay. Follow the tips in INDEX 19 for healthy teeth.

INDEX 19

FOR HEALTHY TEETH AND GUMS

- Between meals, eat few foods or beverages containing sugars or starches. If you do eat them, brush your teeth afterward to reduce risk of tooth decay.
- Brush at least twice a day and floss daily. Use fluoride toothpaste.
- Ask your dentist or health care provider about the need for supplemental fluoride, or dental sealants, especially for children and if your drinking water is not fluoridated.

INDEX 20

MAJOR SOURCES* OF ADDED SUGARS IN THE UNITED STATES

- Soft drinks
- Cakes, cookies, pies
- Fruitades and drinks such as fruit punch and lemonade
- Dairy desserts such as ice cream
- Candy

- All kinds, except diet or sugar-free

Added sugars

Added sugars are sugars and syrups added to foods in processing or preparation, not the naturally occurring sugars in foods like fruit or milk. The body cannot tell the difference between naturally occurring and added sugars because they are identical chemically. Foods containing added sugars provide calories, but may have few vitamins and minerals. In the United States, the number one source of added sugars is nondiet soft drinks (soda or pop). Sweets and candies, cakes and cookies, and fruit drinks and fruitades are also major sources of added sugars.

Intake of a lot of foods high in added sugars, like soft drinks, is of concern. Consuming excess calories from these foods may contribute to weight gain or lower consumption of more nutritious foods. Use INDEX 20 to identify the most commonly eaten foods that are high in added sugars (unless they are labeled "sugar free" or "diet"). Limit your use of these beverages and foods. Drink water to quench your thirst, and offer it to children.

Some foods with added sugars, like chocolate milk, presweetened cereals, and sweetened canned fruits, also are high in vitamins and minerals. These foods may provide extra calories along with the nutrients and are fine if you need the extra calories.

The Nutrition Facts Label gives the content of sugars from all sources (naturally occurring sugars plus added sugars, if any). You can use the Nutrition Facts Label to compare the amount of total sugars among similar products. To find out if sugars have been added, you also need to look at the food label ingredient list. Use INDEX 21 to identify names of some added sugars.

INDEX 21

NAMES FOR ADDED SUGARS THAT APPEAR ON FOOD LABELS

A food is likely to be high in sugars if one of these names appears first or second in the ingredient list, or if several names are listed.

Brown sugar
Corn sweetener
Corn syrup
Dextrose
Fructose
Fruit juice concentrate
Glucose
High-fructose corn syrup
Honey Invert sugar
Lactose
Malt syrup
Maltose
Molasses
Raw sugar
Sucrose
Syrup
Table sugar

Sugar substitutes

Sugar substitutes such as saccharin, aspartame, acesulfame potassium, and sucralose are extremely low in calories. Some people find them useful if they want a sweet taste without the calories. Some foods that contain sugar substitutes, however, still have calories. Unless you reduce the total calories you eat or increase your physical activity, using sugar substitutes will not cause you to lose weight.

Sugars and other health issues

Behavior. Intake of sugars does not appear to affect children's behavior patterns or their ability to learn. Many scientific studies conclude that sugars do not cause hyperactivity in children.

Weight control. Foods that are high in sugars but low in essential nutrients primarily contribute calories to the diet. When you take in extra calories and don't offset them by increasing your physical activity, you will gain weight. As you aim for a healthy weight and fitness, keep an eye on portion size for all foods and beverages, not only those high in sugars. See INDEX 3.

Choose sensibly to limit your intake of beverages and foods that are high in added sugars.

Get most of your calories from grains (especially whole grains), fruits and vegetables, low-fat or non-fat dairy products, and lean meats or meat substitutes.

Take care not to let soft drinks or other sweets crowd out other foods you need to maintain health, such as low-fat milk or other good sources of calcium.

Follow the simple tips listed in INDEX 19 to keep your teeth and gums healthy.

Drink water often.

Choose and prepare foods with less salt

Many people can reduce their chances of developing high blood pressure by consuming less salt. Several other steps can also help keep your blood pressure in the healthy range (see INDEX 22). In the body, sodium—which you get mainly from salt—plays an essential role in regulating fluids and blood pressure. Many studies in diverse populations have shown that a high sodium intake is associated with higher blood pressure.

There is no way to tell who might develop high blood pressure from eating too much salt. However, consuming less salt or sodium is not harmful and can be recommended for the healthy, normal person (see INDEX 23).

At present, the firmest link between salt intake and health relates to blood pressure. High salt intake also increases the amount of calcium excreted in the urine. Eating less salt may decrease the loss of calcium from bone. Loss of too much calcium from bone increases the risk of osteoporosis and bone fractures.

INDEX 22

STEPS THAT MAY HELP KEEP BLOOD PRESSURE IN A HEALTHY RANGE

- Choose and prepare foods with less salt.

- Aim for a healthy weight: blood pressure increases with increases in body weight and decreases when excess weight is reduced.
- Increase physical activity: it helps lower blood pressure, reduce risk of other chronic diseases, and manage weight.
- Eat fruits and vegetables. They are naturally low in salt and calories. They are also rich in potassium (see INDEX 12), which may help decrease blood pressure.
- If you drink alcoholic beverages, do so in moderation. Excessive alcohol consumption has been associated with high blood pressure.

INDEX 23

IS LOWERING SALT INTAKE SAFE?

- Eating too little salt is not generally a concern for healthy people. If you are being treated for a chronic health problem, ask your doctor about whether it is safe for you to reduce your salt intake.
- Some table salt is fortified with iodine. If you use table salt to meet your need for iodine, a small amount—about ¼ teaspoon of iodized salt—provides more than half the daily iodine allowance.
- Your body can adjust to prevent too much sodium loss when you exercise heavily or when it is very hot. However, if you plan to reduce your salt intake and you exercise vigorously, it is sensible to decrease gradually the amount of salt you consume.

Salt is found mainly in processed and prepared foods

Salt (sodium chloride) is the main source of sodium in foods (see INDEX 24). Only small amounts of salt occur naturally in foods. Most of the salt you eat comes from foods that have salt added during food processing or during preparation in a restaurant or at home. Some recipes include table salt or a salty broth or sauce, and some cooking styles call for adding a very salty seasoning such as soy sauce. Not all foods with added salt taste salty. Some people add salt or a salty seasoning to their food at the table. Your preference for salt may decrease if you gradually add smaller amounts of salt or salty seasonings to your food over a period of time.

Aim for a moderate sodium intake

Most people consume too much salt, so moderate your salt intake. Healthy children and adults need to consume only small amounts of salt to meet their sodium needs—less than ¼ teaspoon of salt daily. The Nutrition Facts Label lists a Daily Value of 2,400 mg of sodium per day. This is the amount of sodium in about 1 teaspoon of salt. See INDEX 25 for helpful hints on how to keep your sodium intake moderate.

INDEX 24

Salt Versus Sodium

- Salt contains sodium. Sodium is a substance that affects blood pressure.
- The best way to cut back on sodium is to cut back on salt and salty foods and seasonings.
- When reading a Nutrition Facts Label, look for the sodium content. Foods that are low in sodium (less than 5% of the Daily Value or DV) are low in salt.

INDEX 25

Ways To Decrease Your Salt Intake

At the Store

- Choose fresh, plain frozen, or canned vegetables without added salt most often—they're low in salt.
- Choose fresh or frozen fish, shellfish, poultry, and meat most often. They are lower in salt than most canned and processed forms.
- Read the Nutrition Facts Label to compare the amount of sodium in processed foods— such as frozen dinners, packaged mixes, cereals, cheese, breads, soups, salad dressings, and sauces. The amount in different types and brands often varies widely.

- Look for labels that say "low-sodium." They contain 140 mg (about 5% of the Daily Value) or less of sodium per serving.
- Ask your grocer or supermarket to offer more low sodium foods. Cooking and Eating at Home
- If you salt foods in cooking or at the table, add small amounts. Learn to use spices and herbs, rather than salt, to enhance the flavor of food.
- Go easy on condiments such as soy sauce, ketchup, mustard, pickles, and olives—they can add a lot of salt to your food.
- Leave the salt shaker in a cupboard.
- Eating Out
- Choose plain foods like grilled or roasted entrees, baked potatoes, and salad with oil and vinegar. Batter-fried foods tend to be high in salt, as do combination dishes like stews or pasta with sauce.
- Ask to have no salt added when the food is prepared.

Any Time

- Choose fruits and vegetables often.
- Drink water freely. It is usually very low in sodium. Check the label on bottled water for sodium content.

Choose sensibly to moderate your salt intake.

Choose fruits and vegetables often. They contain very little salt unless it is added in processing.

Read the Nutrition Facts Label to compare and help identify foods lower in sodium—especially prepared foods.

Use herbs, spices, and fruits to flavor food, and cut the amount of salty seasonings by half.

If you eat restaurant foods or fast foods, choose those that are prepared with only moderated amounts of salt or salty flavorings.

If you drink alcoholic beverages, do so in moderation

Alcoholic beverages supply calories but few nutrients. Alcoholic beverages are harmful when consumed in excess, and some people should not drink at all. Excess alcohol alters judgment and can lead to dependency and a great many other serious health problems. Taking more than one drink per day for women or two drinks per day for men (see INDEX 26) can raise the risk for motor vehicle crashes, other injuries, high blood pressure, stroke, violence, suicide, and certain types of cancer. Even one drink per day can slightly raise the risk of breast cancer. Alcohol consumption during pregnancy increases risk of birth defects. Too much alcohol may cause social and psychological problems, cirrhosis of the liver, inflammation of the pancreas, and damage to the brain and heart. Heavy drinkers also are at risk of malnutrition because alcohol contains calories that may substitute for those in nutritious foods. If adults choose to drink alcoholic beverages, they should consume them only in moderation (see INDEX 26)—and with meals to slow alcohol absorption.

INDEX 26

WHAT IS DRINKING IN MODERATION?

Moderation is defined as no more than one drink per day for women and no more than two drinks per day for men. This limit is based on differences between the sexes in both weight and metabolism.

Count as a drink—
12 ounces of regular beer (150 calories)
5 ounces of wine (100 calories)
1.5 ounces of 80-proof distilled spirits (100 calories)
NOTE: Even moderate drinking provides extra calories.

Drinking in moderation may lower risk for coronary heart disease, mainly among men over age 45 and women over age 55. However, there are other factors that reduce the risk of heart disease, including a healthy diet, physical activity, avoidance of smoking, and maintenance of a healthy weight.

Moderate consumption provides little, if any, health benefit for younger people. Risk of alcohol abuse increases when drinking starts at an early age. Some studies suggest that older people may become more sensitive to the effects of alcohol as they age.

Who should not drink?

Some people should not drink alcoholic beverages at all. These include:

Children and adolescents.

Individuals of any age who cannot restrict their drinking to moderate levels. This is a special concern for recovering alcoholics, problem drinkers, and people whose family members have alcohol problems.

Women who may become pregnant or who are pregnant. A safe level of alcohol intake has not been established for women at any time during pregnancy, including the first few weeks. Major birth defects, including fetal alcohol syndrome, can be caused by heavy drinking by the pregnant mother. Other fetal alcohol effects may occur at lower levels.

Individuals who plan to drive, operate machinery, or take part in other activities that require attention, skill, or coordination. Most people retain some alcohol in the blood up to 2 to 3 hours after a single drink.

Individuals taking prescription or over-the-counter medications that can interact with alcohol. Alcohol alters the effectiveness or toxicity of many medications, and some medications may increase blood alcohol levels. If you take medications, ask your health care provider for advice about alcohol intake, especially if you are an older adult.

If you choose to drink alcoholic beverages, do so sensibly, and in moderation.

Limit intake to one drink per day for women or two per day for men, and take with meals to slow alcohol absorption.

Avoid drinking before or when driving, or whenever it puts you or others at risk.

CHAPTER 3

HEALTHY EATING

Antioxidants & Free Radicals

Antioxidants help to protect the body from damage by free radicals. Free radicals are produced in the body because of exercise, pollution, poor diet and smoking. They can attack the blood vessels and increase the risk of heart disease, stroke or cancer. The major antioxidants include vitamins A (beta carotene) C, E, selenium, manganese, zinc, lycopene, lutein and flavonoids and can be found in the following:

Antioxidants	**Food or drink**
Vitamin A/ ß-carotene	Liver, dairy products, eggs, carrots, squash, sweet potatoes, pumpkin, green leafy vegetables, apricots, cantaloupe melon
Vitamin C	Green leafy vegetables, potatoes, cantaloupe melon, citrus fruits, strawberries, blackcurrants, kiwi fruit, mangoes, tomatoes, peppers, white bread
Vitamin E	Vegetable oil, liver, green leafy vegetables, dairy foods, wholegrains, nuts and seeds
Selenium	Seafood, meat, grains, vegetables
Manganese	Nuts, dried fruit, cereals, grains, tea
Zinc	Meat, seafood, fish, poultry, green vegetables
Lycopene and lutein	Tomatoes
Flavonoids	Red wine, grapes, tea, onions

Some antioxidant vitamins (particularly Vitamin C), are destroyed by heat, light and air and leach into cooking water. To look after the vitamins and minerals in your food, try using alternative cooking methods such as steaming, quick stir frying or microwave instead of boiling

Keep a store of frozen fruits and vegetables for when you can't find time to buy fresh. They are just as good as fresh in many ways as they are picked and frozen on the same day and most of the nutritional value is maintained. Tinned fruit and vegetables generally have a lower vitamin and mineral content as a result of processing. Check the salt content of tinned foods and choose those that are vacuum-packed with no salt added

Eat raw fruit and vegetables as snacks or in salads. Fruit makes a great, high carbohydrate, low fat, nutrient dense snack. Vegetables can add bulk to meals which is likely to increase feelings of fullness and help reduce snacking on high fat food between meals

Scientific studies into the effects of vitamins and minerals on the risk of heart disease and cancer continue. Most studies have shown a decreased risk of these diseases in people who have higher intakes of fruit and vegetables

Eat 5 or more portions of fruit and vegetables every day. A portion is equal to: one apple/banana/nectarine/peach/pear, two smaller fruits, e.g. kiwi/plums, a large slice of melon/pineapple, a small glass of fruit juice, 2-3 tablespoons of cooked vegetables or a dessert bowl of salad

It is currently not known how much of particular vitamins and minerals are needed to reduce the risk of disease, so mega-dosing on supplements of vitamins and minerals is not justified. Following a healthy diet with a variety of foods is the safest way to ensure a good balance

Supplements can lead to rebound deficiency (eg vitamin C), vitamin A is toxic in large doses and taking too much of a particular vitamin or mineral can upset the balance of other vitamins and minerals within the body

** This fact sheet provides you with basic information about healthy eating. It is not a substitute for medical or dietetic advice and you should contact your GP for further information

Food & diet

There are a wealth of popular food diets available today so how do you choose the right one for you? Do you need to follow any specific popular diet at all? Surely it is all about eating a wide range of foods in the right balance and getting active? Read on to find out more!

Very Low Calorie Diet (VLCD)

Excessive lowering of total daily calorie intake. This will cause drastic initial weight loss, which comes mainly come from loss of glycogen and water. Lean tissue can be lost in the long term and this is likely to affect metabolic rate and hinder subsequent successful weight control. Prolonged periods on this diet may result in nutritional deficiencies. Many people who follow these diets end up putting the weight back on

Calorie Counting

Based on counting the number of calories eaten throughout the day. It is often an effective way to lose weight but does not take into account how much fat, protein and carbohydrate is eaten or whether it is nutritionally adequate. It can be very time consuming to calculate and problems can arise when eating out!

Food Combining

This diet is based on not mixing different foods together at the same meal, ie carbohydrate and protein. The diet encourages you to eat plenty of fruit and vegetables. Weight losses are more likely to be based on food restriction rather than anything to do with the splitting of foods. This diet often advises against intake of dairy products and or beans and pulses (they just happen to be a good source of both protein and carbohydrate). People on this type of diet are likely to have lower intakes of calcium, vitamin D and Vitamin B12. Difficult to follow for active people or when eating out

Slimming Clubs

There are various approaches. Some clubs use a point system, others split foods into those that can be eaten on certain days. Most members are given a plan to follow and are weighed weekly. For some people the group support they offer is essential and it gives them the sense of 'I am not alone', while others may find it less inviting. The weekly sessions can work out to be quite expensive over a period of time

Meal Replacement Diet

This involves the substitution of one of more meals during the day with either a calorie controlled shake, soup or cereal bar. The diet generally has a fixed number of calories a day that the dieter must follow. This diet does not teach you how to eat healthily and can be very monotonous. It does not particularly help people adopt a new approach and relapse is quite high

The Atkins Diet

Probably the diet of the millennium so far! Advocated by famous stars such as Jennifer Aniston and Julia Roberts it is based on a high protein low carbohydrate intake. Weight loss is reflective of the restriction in calories rather than the elimination of essential food groups. The diet is low in fruit and vegetables and under 100g carbohydrate daily. Having insufficient carbohydrate in your diet initiates the body to start burning off fatty acids. Weakness, nausea, increased headaches, dizziness and constipation may result.

If the diet is followed for a prolonged period of time, ketones are released into the bloodstream, which causes the classic 'alcoholic breath'. High protein diets are usually high in saturated fat, which is linked to the lifestyle diseases obesity and heart disease

** This fact sheet provides you with basic information about healthy eating. It is not a substitute for medical or dietetic advice and you should contact your GP for further information

Vegan : diet information

Vegans avoid all foods of animal origin and their diet generally includes vegetables, vegetable oils, cereals, pulses such as beans and lentils, nuts, fruit and seeds. There is an increased risk of nutritional deficiency if a wide variety of foods in appropriate combinations are not included.

- A vegan diet can be healthy and balanced. It has been shown that there is a lower incidence of heart disease, some cancers, diabetes, high blood pressure, obesity, diabetes and gallstones among vegans. This is probably not solely to do with their dietary regime since vegans adopt many other changes in lifestyle eg they do not usually smoke
- Vegan diets are not necessarily low in protein provided a wide variety of plant protein sources are combined. Individual plant foods do not contain all the essential amino acids the body needs. Foods need to be combined eg grains with pulses, to ensure a complete supply of all the amino acids needed. This is called protein complementing
- Beans on toast, peanut butter sandwich, rice with beans and peas, bean casserole with rice, lentils with bread and dhal and rice are all great choices to help ensure an adequate protein intake
- Use monounsaturated fats for cooking e.g. rapeseed oil, groundnut oil, olive oil or spread. These types of fat can help to protect the heart. Keep total fat intake low as it is the fat in the diet that is most likely to lead to weight gain. Check product labels to see whether foods are less than one third of energy from fat, if they are, then they are lower fat foods
- Meals should be based around starchy foods and include a wide variety, e.g. bread, cereals, pasta, rice, potatoes, as well as other good carbohydrate sources such as peas, beans and pulses, fruit and root vegetables and soya products
- Include at least five portions of fruit and vegetables every day. Choose ones of different colours and varieties. This will help provide a balance of the antioxidants vitamins A, C, E, selenium, lycopene and flavonoids
- Vegans are at high risk of vitamin B12 deficiency as this vitamin is mostly found in animal products. Other sources include yeast extract, some vegetable stocks, textured vegetable protein, fortified soya milk, fortified breakfast cereals, fortified soya mince and chunks.

Nutritional supplements may be necessary in some cases

- Vegans may be at risk of calcium deficiency as they do not eat dairy products. They should regularly include alternative calcium containing foods such as fortified soya milk and products, beans, green leafy vegetables, bread, oranges, apricots and dried fruit in their diet
- Vegans are also at an increased risk of iron deficiency as the main sources of iron are found in animal products such as red meat. Vegans should include alternative food sources of iron on a daily basis, e.g. beans, pulses, fortified cereals and bread, green leafy vegetables, tofu, soya products, nuts and seeds. If a food or drink containing vitamin C is eaten with these plant foods e.g. orange juice with cereal, then iron absorption is likely to be increased
- Vegan diets can have low levels of zinc so ensure you include a wide variety of zinc containing foods on a daily basis, e.g. pulses, nuts, seeds and wholegrain cereals
- The UK National Food Guide, the Balance of Good Health is appropriate for vegans to follow. Vegans should try to have about half of their food from the bread group a third from the vegetable and fruit group and a sixth from the 'alternatives' group

** This fact sheet provides you with basic information about healthy eating. It is not a substitute for medical or dietetic advice and you should contact your GP for further information

Vegetarian : food information

There are types of vegetarian diets and you will need to select the information relevant to you according to the eating plan you follow. The types we refer to are:

- Semi or demi vegetarians exclude red meat but still eat fish and other animal products
- Lacto ovo vegetarians exclude all meat, fish and poultry but still eat dairy products and eggs
- Lacto vegetarians exclude all meat, fish, poultry and eggs but still include dairy products

Vegetarian diets, like all diets, need to be planned appropriately to be nutritionally adequate. Having a vegetarian style of eating does not necessarily mean that your diet is healthier. You still need to monitor your fat intake and ensure you are eating the right choice of food to give you adequate carbohydrate, vitamins and minerals

Studies have shown that a vegetarian diet reduces your risk for several common chronic degenerative diseases and conditions, including obesity, coronary artery disease, hypertension, diabetes mellitus, gallstones and some types of cancer

If you plan your diet carefully you are likely to get all the protein you need from plant based foods alone. Individual plant foods do not contain all the amino acids the body needs and so it is vital to eat a wide variety of foods and combine them together. Combining grains with pulses can lead to a higher quality of protein and this is called protein complementing.

- Soya products, eggs, milk, cheese and yoghurt contain all the amino acids the body needs
- Beans on toast, peanut butter sandwiches, rice with peas or beans, potatoes with egg or cheese, bean casserole with rice, pasta with cheese, rice and milk pudding and cereals with milk are all great options for complete protein
- Generally, vegetarians have a lower intake of saturated fat but you still need to be careful about your total fat intake. Reading food labels can help. For a food to be considered a low fat choice, no more than 35% of its energy should come from fat. Full fat dairy products and cheese all contain saturated fat. Choose semi skimmed milk, reduced fat cheese, use less of a full fat cheese by grating it rather than cutting off chunks and choose low fat yoghurts
- Use rapeseed oil, groundnut oil or olive oil or spread for cooking as this provides monounsaturated fat, which can help to reduce LDL (bad) cholesterol. Keep your total fat intake low as all fat contains 9kcal per gramme and can contribute to weight gain
- Choose a wide variety of carbohydrate foods and base your meals around bread, cereals, pasta, potatoes, rice,

peas, beans, pulses, lentils, milk and dairy products, soya products, bagels, crumpets, muffins, tea cakes and hot cross buns. Choose wholegrain foods wherever possible to increase your total nutrient and fibre intake

- Choose a wide variety of fruit and vegetables to obtain a balance of antioxidant vitamins and minerals; vitamins A, C, E, lycopene, beta carotene and selenium
- If you avoid eating red meat, poultry and fish, which are good sources of iron, ensure you replace these with other good sources of iron in the diet. Peas, beans, pulses, green leafy vegetables, dried fruit, fortified cereals and bread are all alternative sources of iron. Include a source of vitamin C with these foods, such as orange juice, to increase the iron absorption
- Unless you are vegan, you are likely to include milk and milk products in your diet, which may provide adequate calcium. If you don't have these foods ensure you include other food sources of calcium, eg fortified soya products, bread, green leafy vegetables, beans, apricots and oranges
- If you include milk and eggs in your diet you should have an adequate intake of vitamin B12, which is needed for the formation of blood cells. Alternative sources include yeast extract, some vegetable stocks, textured vegetable protein, fortified soya milk and breakfast cereals
- The UK National Food Guide, the Balance of Good Health still applies to vegetarian diets. Try to make up half of your plate with foods from the bread, rice, cereals and pasta group, a third from the vegetables and fruit group and a sixth from the meat, fish and alternative food group
- A label that says "suitable for vegetarians" does not mean that it will be nutritionally balanced

Healthy Eating : the balance of good health

What is healthy eating? Many people see some foods as 'good' and some foods as 'bad' and feel they are helping their health when they are eating 'good' foods and not when eating 'bad'. Healthy eating is all about achieving a balanced diet and to achieve this you should eat a variety of foods in moderation. The problem is that your idea of variety and moderation is probably very different to someone else!

Healthy eating can be achieved by following the Balance of Good Health (BOGH). This is a visual representation of how to achieve a balanced diet and is the UK National Food Guide :

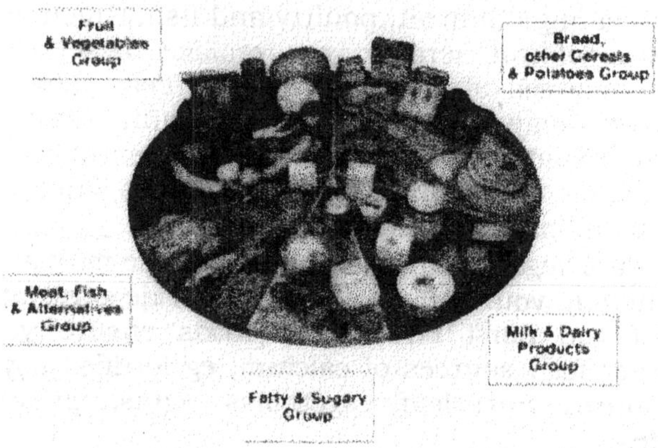

- The BOGH shows you that no food is bad and all food can play a part in a healthy balanced diet. It encourages you to eat a variety of foods from all the food groups meaning that you don't need to deprive yourself of any of your favourite foods
- The BOGH helps to ensure that all your nutritional requirements are met
- The BOGH gives you a guide as to how many portions of food from the different food groups you should eat daily.

The basic food groups

There are five basic food groups :

- Bread, other cereals and potatoes (5-14 portions)
- Milk and dairy products (2 - 3 portions)
- Fruit and vegetables (5 or more portions)
- Meat, fish and alternatives(2- 3 portions)
- Foods containing fat. Foods containing sugar (keep these to minimum)

Contrary to some of the popular diets around today, protein foods should not be eaten in large quantities. Your meals and snacks should be based on starchy carbohydrate foods such as potato, rice, pasta and bread and plenty of fruit and vegetables

The BOGH is appropriate for everyone except for children under the age of 2. This pattern of eating can be introduced into the diet of children between 2-5 years old

The BOGH is suitable for vegetarians, is flexible and uses readily available foods

The BOGH can be adapted for all international foods/diets eg Chinese, Asian, Caribbean

Minerals

All living cells rely on minerals to ensure proper function and structure. They occur naturally as elements in the ground, following millions of years of erosion and breakdown. Particles are assimilated during plant growth and eventually find their way into our bodies through the food chain.

In the human body; minerals function as coenzymes. Coenzymes enable the human body to perform basic functions such as; the production of energy; healthy growth and healing; and assimilation of vitamins and other nutrients by the body.

The body's structure relies on minerals to ensure; muscle tone (including that of the cardiovascular system); healthy functioning of nerves; correct composition of body fluids; and the formation of healthy blood and bones.

Do they have a natural grouping?

There are two distinct groupings;

Macrominerals Calcium, Magnesium, Sodium, Potassium, and Phosphorus

Needed in greater quantities than the trace minerals.

Microminerals Boron, Chromium, Copper, Iodine, Iron, Manganese, Molybdenum, Selenium, Silicon, Sulphur Vanadium and Zinc

Much smaller quantities of these minerals are required by the body.

Once they are in the body, minerals all compete to be absorbed. Certain combinations may hinder and even prevent absorption of each other. Once they have been absorbed, they are carried in the blood to the cells, then carried across the cell membrane in a form that allows the cells to utilise them.

Supplements : vitamins & minerals

What do we mean by supplements? Vitamins and minerals are essential for good health. A lack of a particular vitamin or mineral can lead to a deficiency disease. We have some basic information and facts for you:

- Over 45% of households bought nutrition supplements in the UK last year (2001); £350 million was spent on supplementation and is still rising. Vitamin C is the top selling supplement in the UK
- Supplements are powerfully promoted as a way of optimising health and helping to treat certain conditions. Good health and decreasing your risk of disease is still dependent on achieving a healthy, balanced diet and including a wide variety of foods as part of an active lifestyle
- Supplements contain concentrated amounts of vitamins and minerals and are available in tablets, capsules, powders and liquids. They are not a substitute for a healthy diet and taking a supplement does not make a poor diet better
- Supplements may be taken as single vitamins, e.g. vitamin C, or as combinations such as selenium ACE or multivitamins and multiminerals. You can also buy natural oils, such as fish oils which contain omega 3 fats, which can help to protect against heart disease. Herbal remedies and natural substances promoted for their health enhancing effects, e.g. Royal Jelly are also available
- Scientific studies into the effects of different nutrients on the risk of cancer and heart disease continue. Many studies have looked at the effects of eating more fruit and vegetables, which have been shown to reduce the

risk of both of these diseases

- Fruit and vegetables contain antioxidant vitamins and minerals, e.g. Vitamins A, C, E and selenium, and other antioxidants may be found in certain foods such as phyto oestrogens in soya, lycopene in tomatoes and flavonoids in tea and red wine
- It is not currently known whether individual vitamins and minerals help to protect the body against disease or whether it is a combination of nutrients, such as those found within foods such as fruit and vegetables
- Megadoses of individual vitamins are not currently justified by scientific evidence and may even be harmful. Vitamin A is toxic in large doses as it is stored in body fat. Cod liver oil, Evening Primrose Oil, multivitamins and minerals and selenium A, C, E all contain vitamin A and many people take combinations of these supplements without realising the potential harm
- If you take too much of one particular vitamin or mineral it can upset the balance of other vitamins and minerals within the body
- If large doses of vitamin C are taken, i.e. 500mg to 1000mg when the requirement for adults is only 40mg, the body is only able to absorb a small amount and the rest is passed out though the urine. Rebound deficiency can occur when large doses are suddenly stopped. The body gets used to a higher level of vitamin C and if the supplement is stopped the body can become deficient in vitamin C
- Look at your diet first and make changes to include a range of nutrient dense foods. Eat plenty of fruit and vegetables, wholegrains, lean meat, fish, beans, pulses and low fat dairy products. If you suspect that you need to increase your intake of any particular vitamin and mineral, positively include foods rich in that particular vitamin or mineral regularly in your diet
- Taking iron supplements without medical supervision is not advisable as it may cover up a more serious condition. Too much iron can be damaging to the body. Iron can be obtained from foods such as offal, red meat, poultry, fish, peas, beans, pulses, green leafy vegetables, wholegrain foods and fortified cereals. It is

wise to include these foods rather than relying on a supplement

- You may need to consider taking a supplement if you are;
- Planning to get pregnant
- Eating haphazardly and grabbing foods without thought
- On a reducing diet and cutting daily calories
- Ill or recovering from an illness
- A vegan
- Suffering from a food allergy or intolerance
- Following a fad diet which excludes total food groups

Vitamins

Vitamins and minerals are essential for life. As well as helping to regulate our metabolism they play a key role in the complex biochemical processes that give us energy from the breakdown of food that we ingest. Apart from Vitamin D, which can be made with the aid of sunlight, you will derive everything else from the food you eat.

They can be either water-soluble (Vitamins B and C), or oil-soluble (Vitamins A, D, E and K). Water-soluble cannot be stored in our bodies, whereas oil-soluble are stored in fatty tissue and the liver. Our bodies should therefore be provided with water-soluble ones daily.

How do we get them?

Vitamins and minerals must be taken in appropriate quantities so as not to upset the body's natural balance. Ideally, these should come from fresh and healthy foods.

However, sometimes we need to use supplements in a tablet, powder or liquid form. These should not be considered as a simple alternative to a good healthy balanced diet. If supplements must be taken, if possible, they should be natural whole food supplements (derived from food sources), as opposed to synthetic supplements (produced as chemicals in laboratories). All supplements work best when they are combined with food and medical studies show that oil-soluble vitamins should be taken before meals, water-soluble after.

On the following pages, with the help of the Health Food Manufacturers Association (HFMA), we have set out the basic information about what they are important for, their sources, effects any deficiency may cause and additional information - where appropriate. This is not an exhaustive guide but may help you to understand the differences between all the different types.

Vitamin A : guide (Beta-Carotene)

Beta Carotene, or Vitamin A, can be obtained from either animal or vegetable sources. The animal form is divided between retinol and dehydroretinol whereas the vegetable beta-carotene can be split into four very potent groups - alpha-carotene, beta-carotene, gamma-carotene and crypto-carotene. With enough beta-carotene available in the body, the body can manufacture its own.

Important for :Utilizing protein; formation of bones and teeth; new cell growth; maintenance and repair of epithelial tissue (skin and mucous membranes of the mouth, nose, throat and lungs); aiding protection against airborne infections (flu and colds).

Sources :Green and yellow fruits and vegetables (e.g. apricots; asparagus; broccoli; carrots; garlic; papayas; peaches; pumpkin; red peppers; spinach; squash; turnip greens and watercress). Animal livers and fish liver oils.

Herbs (e.g. alfalfa; burdock root; cayenne; fennel; hops; kelp; lemongrass; paprika; parsley; peppermint; raspberry leaf; rosehips; sage and violet leaves).

Possible deficiency symptoms : Night blindness; dryness of the eyes; increased susceptibility to illness or infection such as colds; rough or dry skin; acne; poor growth; loss of smell and/or appetite; insomnia; and teeth and gum problems.

Hinders maximum absorption : Antibiotics, alcohol and coffee may impede absorption by the body

Additional Information : Acts as an antioxidant, helping to protect cells from disease and best taken with food for maximum absorption.

A class of compounds related to vitamin A is classified as Carotenoids. The most commonly known is Beta-carotene, which is converted into vitamin A in the liver. Taking too much Beta-carotene may turn your skin an orangey-yellow colour but is not harmful.

Overdosing for lengthy periods can be toxic to the liver. Overdosing cannot occur with Beta-carotene.

Vitamin B1 (Thiamin) : guide

Thiamine, or Vitamin B1, is important for nervous system function, musculature and cardiovascular health, as well as for normal growth and development. The essential co-enzyme also aids in metabolizing carbohydrates, and it helps to regulate the appetite. Can be lost in cooking and food preparation so supplements are advised :

Important for :Enhancing the body's ability to generate energy through the metabolic cycle; digestion of carbohydrates due to increased production of hydrochloric acid; muscle tone in the intestines, heart and lungs; optimising brain functions; growth.

Sources : The richest sources are; brown rice; chicken; egg yolks; fish; liver; peanuts; pork; wheat germ; and whole grains.

Additional sources include; asparagus; broccoli; Brussels sprouts; kelp; nuts; oatmeal; plums; prunes; raisins; and watercress.

Herbs (e.g. alfalfa; bladder-wrack; burdock root; cayenne; chamomile; fennel; fenugreek; hops; nettles; parsley; peppermint; raspberry leaf; rosehips; and sage).

Possible deficiency symptoms : Loss of appetite; constipation; fatigue; irritability; insomnia; forgetfulness; difficulty breathing; heart and gastrointestinal problems; poor co-ordination and concentration; weight loss.

Hinders maximum absorption : Antibiotics, oral contraceptives and diuretics, such as tea and coffee, may decrease the level of thiamine in the body.

Additional Information : High carbohydrate diets need increased amount of thiamine.

Thiamine acts as an antioxidant, protecting against aging, alcohol and smoking.

Vitamin B2 (Riboflavin) : Guide

Vitamin B12 is a member of the B complex group. It contains cobalt, and so is also known as cobalamin. It is exclusively synthesised by bacteria and is found primarily in meat, eggs and dairy products. It's primary functions are in the formation of red blood cells and the maintenence of a healthy nervous system.

Important for :Formation and regeneration of red blood cells, digestion and absorption of foods; carbohydrate and fat metabolism; synthesis of protein; promoting normal growth; increasing energy.

Sources : Richest sources are; brewer's yeast; clams; dairy products; eggs; herring; kidney; liver; mackerel; milk; and seafood.

Herbs (e.g. alfalfa; bladder wrack; hops)

Possible deficiency symptoms : Fatigue; poor appetite; depression; digestive disorders; nervousness; irritability; anaemia.

Hinders maximum absorption : Alcohol and smoking decreases absorption of B-12 by the body.

Additional Information : Deficiency of B-12 can be caused by poor absorption due to digestive disorders.

Vegetarians may need to have natural supplements of B-12, as it is found almost exclusively in animal products.

Riboflavin (Vitamin B2) is manufactured in the body by the intestinal flora and is easily absorbed, although very small quantities are stored, there is a constant need for this vitamin. It is required by the body to use oxygen & metabolism of amino acids, fatty acid

& carbohydrates.

Important for :Formation of red blood cells and antibodies; growth; cell respiration; aiding metabolism of carbohydrates, fats and proteins; facilitating the use of oxygen to maintain healthy skin, nails and hair; absorption of iron; alleviating eye fatigue.

Sources : Richest sources are; cheese; egg yolks; fish; meat; milk; poultry; spinach; whole grains; yoghurt.

Additional sources include; asparagus; avocados; broccoli; Brussels sprouts; currants; greens; kelp; mushrooms; nuts; and watercress.

Herbs (e.g. alfalfa; bladder-wrack; burdock root; cayenne; chamomile; chickweed; fennel; fenugreek; ginseng; horsetail; hops; nettles; oat straw; parsley; peppermint; raspberry leaf; rosehips; and sage).

Possible deficiency symptoms : Cracks and sores on mouth and lips; split nails; inflamed mouth and tongue; itching and burning eyes; insomnia; digestion problems; dermatitis; cataracts.

Hinders maximum absorption : Riboflavin is easily destroyed by antibiotics and alcohol.

Additional Information : Additional Riboflavin acts as an antioxidant, protecting against aging, alcohol and smoking.

Riboflavin should be taken when using oral contraceptives and with increased exercise.

Vitamin B3 (Niacin) : guide

Important for :Improving circulation and reducing cholesterol levels in the blood; maintaining nervous system; metabolising carbohydrates, fats and proteins; increasing production of hydrochloric acid for digestive system; healthy skin; synthesis of sex hormones.

Sources : Found in; beef liver; broccoli; carrots; cheese; corn flour; dates; eggs; fish; milk; peanuts; pork; potatoes; tomatoes; wheat germ; and wheat products.

Herbs; (e.g. alfalfa; burdock root; catnip; cayenne; chamomile; eyebright; fennel; hops; liquorice; nettles; oat straw; parsley; peppermint; raspberry leaf; rosehips; and yellow dock).

Possible deficiency symptoms : Headaches; fatigue; depression; dementia; dizziness; insomnia; aches and pains; irritability; loss of appetite; skin disorders; bad breath; muscular weakness.

Hinders maximum absorption : Tea, coffee and alkaline agents (Baking powder) all prevent maximum absorption by the body.

Additional Information : B3 is absorbed more easily when taken in conjunction with other B-vitamins

Suffers of diabetes, glaucoma, liver disease or ulcers should see a doctor before taking vitamin B3.

Vitamin B5 (Pantohthenic acid) : guide

Important for :Production of adrenal hormones; formation of antibodies; conversion of fats, proteins and carbohydrates into energy; improving resistance to stress; helping vitamin utilization; producing neurotransmitters; prevention of anaemia.

Sources : The richest sources are; beef; brewers yeast; eggs; fresh vegetables; greens; liver; mushrooms; nuts; pork; saltwater fish; whole rye flour; and whole wheat.

Possible deficiency symptoms : Tingling sensations in the hands; painful and burning feet; nausea and headaches; dizzy spells; restlessness.

Hinders maximum absorption : Antibiotics, tea, coffee, contraceptive pills and alcohol all hinder absorption by the body.

Additional Information : May be useful in helping depression and anxiety and are best taken with food.

Known as the 'anti-stress vitamin'

Vitamin B6 : guide

Important for :Synthesis and breakdown of amino acids; producing hydrochloric acid; absorption of fats and protein; aiding formation of antibodies; helping to maintain proper balance of sodium and phosphorus in the body; reducing water retention; synthesizing nucleic acids RNA and DNA (contain genetic instructions for all cell reproduction); nervous system; activating enzymes; healthy skin.

Sources : All foods contain some vitamin B6, the richest sources are; brewer's yeast; carrots; chicken; eggs; fish; meat; peas; spinach; and wheat germ.

Additional sources include; avocado; bananas; beans; broccoli; brown rice; cabbage; corn; potatoes; rice bran; soy beans; and whole grains.

Herbs; including alfalfa; catnip; and oat straw

Possible deficiency symptoms : Anemia; insomnia; nervousness; loss of muscular control; dermatitis; hair loss; depression; tingling sensations.

Hinders maximum absorption : Stress, alcohol, tea, coffee and heat prevent absorption by the body.

Additional Information : Involved in more body functions than virtually any other nutrient.

If you are taking anti-depressants and/or oral contraceptives this may increase the bodies need for B6.

Vitamin C : guide

Probably, the most important of them all, Vitamin C is the most important one to supplement as it is associated with growth, energy, skin condition and resistance to disease - especially colds and flu. This supplement is required in the synthesis of collagen in connective tissue, neurotransmitters, steroid hormones, carnitine, conversion of cholesterol to bile acids and enhances iron bio availability.

Important for :Ensuring healthy bones, teeth and gums; building resistance to infection; tissue growth and repair; production of anti-stress hormones; helping to reduce cholesterol and high blood pressure; protecting against blood clots and bruises; synthesis of collagen; prevention of scurvy; healing wounds and scar tissues.

Sources : Found in citrus fruits and vegetables, rich sources include; asparagus; avocados; blackcurrants; broccoli; Brussels sprouts; cantaloupe melons; dandelions; grapefruit; lemons; mangos; onions; oranges; papayas; green peas; sweet peppers; persimmons; pineapple;

radishes; rosehips; spinach; strawberries; tomatoes; turnip leaves; and watercress.

Herbs (e.g. alfalfa; burdock root; cayenne; chickweed; fennel; fenugreek; hops; peppermint; nettle; oat straw; paprika; parsley; pin needle; raspberry leaf; rosehips; skullcap; violet leaves; and yellow dock).

Possible deficiency symptoms : Susceptibility to colds and infection; soft and bleeding gums; swollen or painful joints; slow-healing wounds and fractures; bruising; lack of energy; loss of appetite; anemia.

Hinders maximum absorption : Alcohol, analgesics, antidepressants, oral contraceptives and steroids may reduce the body's levels of vitamin C. Smoking causes an even higher depletion.

Additional Information : Vitamin C is an antioxidant, which helps to hinder cell damage caused by free radicals.

If pregnant, high doses of vitamin C (>5,000mg) should not be taken.

Vitamin D : guide

Important for :Absorption and utilisation of calcium and phosphorus; normal growth of bones and teeth in children; a properly functioning thyroid; enhancing immunity; maintaining a stable nervous system and normal heart action.

Sources: Found in; fish liver oil; fatty saltwater fish; dairy products and eggs. Also found in; halibut; liver; oatmeal; salmon; sweet potatoes; vegetable oils.

Herbs; (e.g. alfalfa; nettle; and parsley)

Possible deficiency symptoms : Excessive tooth decay; muscular weakness; loss of appetite; insomnia; weight loss.

Hinders maximum absorption : Cholesterol reducing drugs, mineral oils and steroids interfere with the body's absorption of vitamin D.

Additional Information : Vitamin D is obtained both by ingesting and by spontaneous formation in the skin by the sun via a photochemical reaction in the epidermis.

Liver and gallbladder disorders also reduce absorption.

Important for :Slowing cellular aging and damage from oxidation; preventing red blood cell damage and nerve destruction; improving circulation; blood clotting; maintaining healthy muscles and nerves; strengthening capillary walls; healthy skin; preventing anemia;

Sources : Found in; dark green leafy vegetables; greens; nuts; seeds; and whole grains.

Additional sources include; brown rice; cornmeal; eggs; kelp; dessicated liver; milk; oatmeal; soybeans; sweet potatoes; watercress; wheat; and wheat germ. Herbs; (e.g. alfalfa; bladder wrack; dandelion; nettle; oat straw; raspberry leaf; rosehips)

Possible deficiency symptoms :Skin disorders; reduced sexual libido; loss of reproductive drive.

Hinders maximum absorption : Air pollution, contraceptive pills and excessive processed fats and oils can all hinder absorption of vitamin E by the body.

Additional Information : A major antioxidant.

The body requires zinc to maintain a proper level of vitamin E in the bloodstream.

Vitamin K : guide

Important for :Production of prothrombin, for blood clotting; bone formation and repair; conversion of glucose into glycogen for storage; reducing fatigue; increasing resistance to infection;

Sources : The majority of vitamin K is synthesized by bacteria normally present in the intestines.

Found in; asparagus; broccoli; Brussels sprouts; cabbage; cauliflower; dark green leafy vegetables; egg yolks; liver; oatmeal; oats; rye; soybeans; and wheat.

Herbs; including alfalfa; green tea; kelp; nettle; oat straw

Possible deficiency symptoms : Internal bleeding and non-clotting of blood; fatigue; poor healing of wounds.

Hinders maximum absorption : Antibiotics interfere with the body's absorption of vitamin K. This is because they kill the bacteria in the intestines that synthesize the vitamin.

Additional Information: Not necessary to take as supplements in most cases.

Meal Planning

Athletics is becoming increasingly competitive. More and more stress is being placed on how well you perform. To reach your highest potential, all of your body systems must be perfectly tuned. Nothing is more important to your well-being and ability to perform than good nutrition. Eating the right foods helps you maintain desirable body weight, stay physically fit, and establish optimum nerve-muscle reflexes. Without the right foods, even physical conditioning and expert coaching aren't enough to push you to your best. Good nutrition must be a key part of your training program if you are to succeed.

There is no one "miracle food" or supplement that can supply all of your nutritional needs. Certain foods supply mainly proteins, other foods contain vitamins and minerals, and so on. The key to balancing your diet is to combine different foods so that nutrient deficiencies in some foods are made up by nutrient surpluses in others. Eating a variety of foods is the secret.

The nutrients—the proteins, carbohydrates, fats, vitamins, minerals, and water—are teammates that work together to provide good nutrition. Just as each team member carries out different tasks during a game, each nutrient performs specific functions in your body. A lack of just one nutrient is a disadvantage to your body, just as losing a player to the penalty box is a disadvantage for a hockey team. Your body needs all these nutrients all of the time, so the foods you eat should supply them every day.

Just because you are not hungry does not necessarily mean that your body has all the nutrients it needs. You can fill up on foods that contain mostly carbohydrates and fats, but your body still has basic needs for proteins, minerals, and vitamins.

How can you tell if your diet is stacking up? Nutritionists have developed a food-guide system in the shape of a pyramid that can help you rate or evaluate your diet. This guide divides food into five groups on the basis of the nutrients each group provides. By eating the recommended amounts of food from each group daily, you can greatly increase your ability to get all the nutrients your body needs—and that will improve your ability on the playing field.

Here is some additional information about the food groups that can help you improve your diet.

Milk, Yogurt, and Cheese Group (Milk, yogurt, and all types of cheese) Provides calcium. Also contains protein, vitamin A, and riboflavin (B2).

3 servings daily.
1 serving is

- an 8 ounce glass of milk
- 8 ounces of yogurt
- 1 ½ ounces of natural, unprocessed cheese

Meat, Poultry, Fish, Dry Beans, Eggs, and Nuts Group (Beef, pork, lamb, poultry, fish, eggs, dry peas, dry beans, peanuts, peanut butter) Good source of protein. These foods also contain thiamin (B1), riboflavin (B2), niacin, iron, and zinc. 2 to 3 servings daily.

1 serving is

- 3 ounces of lean, cooked meat
- 2 eggs
- 1 cup of cooked dry beans, peas, or lentils
- 4 tablespoons of peanut butter

Vegetable Group (All vegetables—including dark green, deep yellow, and starchy vegetables—and their juices) Provides vitamins and minerals that complement other food sources. Good sources of Vitamin C include tomatoes, broccoli, and brussel sprouts. Good sources of Vitamin A include carrots, broccoli, spinach, greens, pumpkin, and sweet potatoes.

3 to 5 servings daily.
1 serving is

- ½ cup of cooked vegetables
- ½ cup of chopped raw vegetables

- 1 cup of leafy raw vegetables such as lettuce or spinach
- ¾ cup (6 ounces) of juice

Fruit Group (All fruits and their juices) - Good source of many vitamins and minerals. Good sources of vitamin C include citrus fruits and their juices, melons, and strawberries. Apricots are good sources of vitamin A. - 2 to 4 servings daily.

1 serving is

- 1 whole fruit such as a medium apple, banana, or orange
- ½ grapefruit
- ¾ cup (6 ounces) of juice
- ½ cup (4 ounces) of berries
- ½ cup (4 ounces) of cooked or canned fruit
- ¼ cup of dried fruit

Bread, Cereal, Rice, and Pasta Group (All whole-grain and enriched breads and cereals, such as cooked or ready to eat cereals, bread, macaroni, grits, spaghetti, crackers, noodles, and rice) Contributes complex carbohydrates (starch and fiber) and significant amounts of protein, B vitamins, and iron. - 6 to 11 servings daily.

1 serving is

- 1 slice of bread
- ½ hamburger bun or English muffin
- 1 small roll, biscuit, or muffin
- 3 to 4 small or 2 large crackers
- ½ cup cooked cereal, rice, or pasta
- 1 ounce ready-to-eat breakfast cereal

To meet increased energy needs, most teen athletes require more than the minimum number of servings listed. In some cases, a teen athlete may need more than the recommended number of servings. For most athletes, the increased energy should come from the vegetable group and the bread, cereal, rice, and pasta group. Foods in these two groups contain a lot of starch, which is an excellent source of food energy. Athletes who participate in very high levels of physical activity and/or who have the largest body stature will require the highest intake of food energy.

Foods that occupy the smallest area at the top of the Food Guide Pyramid, such as butter, margarine, sweets, and jellies, should be used sparingly. These foods do provide energy and some nutrients. However, go easy on these foods and get your energy from foods that are more nutritious. Your body needs the additional vitamins and minerals to help it use energy. Make this food guide pyramid system the basis of your training table.

Do athletes have special nutrient needs?

Increased physical activity increases some of your food needs. You require more energy, water, and possibly salt (sodium chloride). An athletic teenage boy may need 5,000 calories a day, compared to the 3,000 calories required daily by his nonathletic friends. By taking extra servings of foods from all food groups (particularly breads, cereals, vegetables, and fruits), you can fill this increased energy need.

Water lost through sweating is not easily replaced. Low water-intake during strenuous exercise leads to dehydration, which can lead to fatigue, heatstroke, and death. Replacement water should never be restricted during exercise. If you drink too much water too quickly during increased physical activity, you may become "waterlogged," an unpleasant condition that you may already have experienced. Moderate amounts of cool water taken frequently before, during, and after activity prevent this problem. Six to eight ounces of fluid taken every fifteen to twenty minutes during strenuous activity is about right for most athletes.

Cool water (around 40 to 50 degrees Fahrenheit) is best. Cool water helps absorb body heat, and it empties from the stomach at a faster rate, which allows it to be absorbed into the body more rapidly.

There are many different commercial sports drinks available. They contain varying kinds and amounts of sugars and electrolytes. Whether they offer advantages over plain water depends on the situation. Many times, plain water is all that an athlete needs. When activities last an hour or more, however, some sport drinks may offer advantages both for carbohydrate and electrolyte replacement.

If you use a sport drink, use one that has less than 8% total solids (sugars, electrolytes). More concentrated solutions can delay fluid absorption. Also, avoid drinks that contain fructose as the only source of carbohydrate. Fructose may cause upset stomach. Additionally, fructose must first be converted to glucose before it can be used for energy. This conversion delays its use as an energy source.

Salt needs can be met by increased use of salt on foods. The use of salt tablets is not recommended. Salt tablets can cause stomach cramps. The tablets hold water in the stomach longer and can actually cause water to be pulled back into the intestinal tract and away from body tissues where the water is needed most.

Are high-protein diets necessary for the high-school athlete?

At one time, it was believed that muscle-building exercise greatly increased dietary protein needs. This idea led to the development of special high-protein meals and drinks for athletes. This greatly increased need for protein was exaggerated, but an athlete's need for protein does increase somewhat. Besides muscle-building, aerobic exercise like distance running may also burn some protein for energy. That's why it is important for all athletes to have adequate protein intakes.

However, these increased protein needs can be met quite easily without using protein supplements or consuming high-protein diets. Increasing basic foods to meet your increased energy needs will supply more than enough protein.

Eating high-protein diets or taking protein supplements may prove harmful and may lead to loss of appetite, diarrhea, dehydration, and undue stress on the kidneys. Extra protein is also expensive.

Does the athlete need vitamin or mineral supplements?

Opinions vary. Increased physical activity increases calorie needs. For the body to use these extra calories, you may need greater amounts of nutrients such as riboflavin, thiamin, niacin, and iron. But again, increasing nutritious foods to meet increased energy needs should supply more than enough vitamins and minerals.

Experts agree that the basis of good nutrition is a well-balanced diet and that vitamin supplements are no substitute for it. Excessive amounts of some vitamins (especially vitamins A and D) taken as supplements over a prolonged period have proved harmful, so depend on a well-balanced diet to supply all your vitamin needs.

Some people think that athletes should take potassium supplements. However, including potassium-rich foods such as oranges, bananas, and baked potatoes will supply adequate potassium. Potassium supplements are not necessary.

Iron deficiency can be a problem with some teenage female athletes, particularly during menstruation and for those on self-prescribed weight-reduction diets. However, the female athlete should not self-prescribe iron supplements. She should question her family doctor about this potential problem and her individual need for iron. The doctor may prescribe an iron supplement after a clinical examination.

What should the athlete eat before a game?

Before a game, your digestive processes may be slowed down by your keyed-up emotional state. To allow for this condition, you should eat an easily digestible meal no later than three hours before the contest. Avoid foods that contain substantial amounts of fats or oils. Fats are more slowly digested than other nutrients. Trying to participate with a high-fat meal still in your stomach is a losing proposition. Meals high in starches are better because they are digested more rapidly than fats or oils.

Some athletes like poached eggs, toast, and juice as a light pregame meal. Some prefer breakfast cereal with low-fat milk, toast with just a little jelly, and juice. All-day events such as track meets or basketball and soccer tournaments present special problems. Consuming several high-starch minimeals or snacks, accompanied by ample fluids, is a winning strategy for these situations.

Avoid sugary foods such as candy or honey before a contest. Sweets can cause rapid swings in blood-sugar levels and result in low blood sugar and less energy.

Is carbohydrate loading (also called glycogen loading) recommended for the high school athlete?

The aim of this practice is to increase the amount of glycogen , or animal starch, stored in liver and muscle tissues. The body makes glycogen from extra carbohydrates it has. This stored glycogen can be broken down and used for energy when needed. That's why it's good for athletes to have sufficient glycogen stores in their bodies at the start of an event.

Carbohydrate-loading is practiced by mature athletes who participate in endurance events such as long-distance running and swimming of long duration. To begin, the athlete eats a high-protein, high-fat, low-carbohydrate diet for a few days. While on this diet, the athlete exercises strenuously. This depletes, or lowers, the body's glycogen stores. After the depletion phase and just a few days before the event, the competitor eats a very high-carbohydrate diet (for example, pancakes, rice, and noodles). During this period, the athlete exercises very little. This eating and exercise routine increases the body's stores of glycogen in liver and muscle tissue, so more carbohydrates are available for muscle energy during endurance events. Carbohydrate loading should not be confused with a diet high in carbohydrates, which is recommended for all athletes, including teenagers.

Carbohydrate loading routines have not been thoroughly tested for the rapidly growing high-school athlete. The disadvantages may outweigh the advantages. Events for most high-school athletes are not long enough to exhaust the normal levels of muscle glycogen. Ultra-high tissue levels of glycogen are not necessary for most sport activities. During the high-protein, high-fat phase of carbohydrate loading, even the mature athlete may not perform as well and may feel exhausted. Young athletes find it difficult to practice during this phase. During the final phase, the body retains water and gains weight.

So full-blown carbohydrate loading is probably not in the best interest of the high-school athlete. However, young athletes can ensure adequate glycogen stores by eating more starchy foods and reducing exercise the last twenty-four to forty-eight hours before the event. This very modified form of carbohydrate loading has proved beneficial to some young athletes.

Should teen athletes try to reduce their weight to make special weight categories?

Moderate weight reduction over an extended period of time, together with a balanced diet to ensure sufficient protein, vitamins, and minerals, may be necessary for some athletes to lose excess fat, which has been shown to limit performance. However, severe weight reduction or restriction of normal weight gain is not recommended. Glycogen and water are usually the first materials to be lost by the athlete on a quick weight-loss plan. Losing glycogen or water can be disastrous to performance and health. When you lose glycogen, you lose energy to power muscles. Losing water lessens your body's ability to cool itself, and endurance decreases.

Repeated episodes of starvation and dehydration during growth slow muscle development. Lost muscle growth will not be restored later. So losing weight rapidly or restricting normal weight gain is not good for you.

Eating Practice Every Day

The training period offers you an excellent opportunity to establish sound eating practices that will benefit you on the playing field as well as give you a measure of well-being throughout life.

Make Snacks Count

Chose snacks that contain more than just calories. When you eat out with friends, choose something nutritionally sound, like a cheeseburger with a slice of tomato and lettuce leaf. How many food groups are present in this sandwich? What might you eat along with this sandwich to make an even better snack?

Look for Extra Food Energy

Teenage athletes burn up more calories than non-athletic teens. You can fill this requirement by eating more food from all food groups. Carbohydrates are the most efficient fuel for your body during strenuous exercise. Get most of your extra energy from foods like starchy vegetables and whole grain or enriched bread, cereal, rice, or pasta instead of from fatty foods. For example, on an athlete's plate, a baked potato should get the nod over french fries.

Eat Regularly

Breakfast is especially important because you need food to start the day. Your body begins the day in a low-energy, fasted condition. Teens who eat breakfast score higher on physical fitness tests. Breakfasts can be made up of any combination of nutritious foods that you enjoy eating. Spaghetti and meatballs, together with an orange and a glass of milk, is a nutritionally sound meal for any time of the day-even breakfast!

Check Your Diet Frequently

Spot-check your daily diet at least once a week. Are you eating at least the minimum number of servings from each food group each day? How can you use the food guide pyramid as a tool to make improvements?

Meal Planner

What you eat every day can have a big effect on how you perform. What you eat right before an event can be critical. Wrong choices can be disastrous. Right choices can give you that competitive edge. The Pregame Meal Planner will help you make wise food choices.

While the pregame meal can supply your body with significant amounts of energy, don't expect it to supply all the energy you'll need for the event. You should eat the right kinds of food for several days before the event to charge up your muscles with glycogen. Glycogen is a key energy source your muscles use during most sports activities. Although the pregame meal won't cause large increases in muscle glycogen, it will:

- Help avoid hunger during the event
- Stablize blood-sugar levels and add some food energy to complement existing energy stores of muscle glycogen
- Hydrate the body (supply water to the body's cells)
- Provide a relatively empty stomach at game time
- Prevent gastrointestinal upset or other adverse reactions to food

No one pregame meal is right for every athlete or every event, but some food choices are much smarter than others. General guidelines for individual food selection and meal planning are on the following page. Make sure your pregame meal plans follow these guidelines.

Make sure your pregame meal plans follow these guidelines

- Allow enough time for digestion. Eat the meal at least three hours before an event.
- Choose a meal that's high in starch. Starch is easy to digest and helps steady the levels of blood sugar.
- Consume only moderate amounts of protein. Protein foods take longer to digest than starch. And high-protein meals may lead to increased urine production, which can add to dehydration.
- Limit fats and oils. They take too long to digest.
- Restrict sugary foods. Sweets can cause rapid energy swings in blood sugar levels and result in low blood sugar and less energy.
- Avoid foods and drinks that contain caffeine. Caffeine stimulates the body to increase urine output, which can contribute to dehydration problems, and a full bladder can be very uncomfortable.
- Watch out for foods that produce gas. Certain raw vegetables, fruits, or beans may cause problems for some young athletes. Be aware of the foods that cause you problems, and avoid them just before an event.
- Within these guidelines, chose foods you like to eat.
- Remember to drink plenty of fluids with your pregame meal.

Here are some nutritious pregame meal plans that fit the pregame guidelines. At least three of the five major groups are represented in each meal. These meals are only suggestions. You can probably think up many more that you would like to eat.

Meal 1
Cereal
(avoid highly sweetened cereals)
Banana slices
Milk (low-fat or skim)
Toast/jam
Pineapple juice*
Water

Meal 2
Chicken noodle soup
Crackers
Orange
Low-fat yogurt
Water

Meal 3
Poached Egg
Toast/jam
Milk (low-fat or skim)
Orange juice*
Water

Meal 4
Pancakes (limit butter and syrup)
Applesauce
Milk (low-fat or skim)
Grape juice*
Water

Meal 5
Turkey sandwich/bread and lettuce
Apple
Milk (low-fat or skim)
Tomato juice*
Water

Meal 6
Cottage cheese/peach
Breadsticks
Milk (low-fat or skim)
Apple juice

Water
Meal 7
Spaghetti/tomato sauce
Bread
Milk (low-fat or skim)
Orange juice*
Water
*Juice of your choice, except prune juice

Foods to choose
Pasta
Macaroni, spaghetti, noodles, ravioli (plain or with sauce)
Meats, cheese, and oil add fat to the sauce. Use them sparingly.
Rice Use a sauce low in fat and only as spicy as you can tolerate easily. Or try rice with a little soy sauce flavoring.
Potatoes

Baked, boiled, mashed, but not french fries -limit butter, gravy, or sour cream.

Starchy vegetables

Peas, carrots, winter squash, sweet potatos - Cooked vegetables are more easily digested.

Breads

Rolls, muffins, crackers, quick breads, bagels –Use nutritious, low-fat bread products and spreads.

Cereals

Oatmeal, other hot cereals, cold cereals - Avoid cereals with high sugar content.

Soups

Noodle, rice, vegetable, clear broth, bouillon, or consomme
Choose low-fat soups. Eating large portions of chilli, split pea, or bean soups may lead to digestive problems for some athletes.

Pancakes - Limit butter and syrup.

Fruits, fruit juices - Use any juice or cooked fruit except prune. Oranges, bananas, and peeled apples are easily digested raw fruits. You may wish to dilute juices, especially in hot weather. Try hot cider or juice during cold weather.

Milk products

Low-fat milk, low-fat yogurt, low-fat cottage cheese, low-fat cheeses, puddings, "shakes" made with low-fat milk or yogurt and fruit and/or juice - Avoid high-fat milk products before games.

Liquid meals in a can Though not a substitute for solid foods in the daily diet, liquid meals are convenient for occasional pregame use. You can make liquid meals at home using the following recipe, which makes about one quart:

½ cup of water
½ cup of nonfat dry milk
¼ cup of sugar
3 cups of skim milk
Flavor with a teaspoon of vanilla or cherry extract.
Foods to avoid

Candy, sugar, honey - After an initial rise, your blood-sugar level can actually drop below normal, resulting in a sudden feeling of tiredness or fatigue.

Tea, coffee, chocolate, cola - Caffeine consumption leads to dehydration.

Fried foods, high-fat meats, fats, oils, gravies, sour cream, etc. - Fat digests slowly and therefore stays in the stomach longer.

Some raw fruits, vegetables, popcorn, nuts, dry beans and peas - Some of these foods may cause gas and/or an uncomfortable feeling of fullness during the game. An athlete needs to avoid the foods that give him or her problems.

Any new food Don't experiment with new foods right before an event. If you experience any adverse reactions, your body has little time to recover.

Fruit-flavored drinks - Many drinks contain little fruit juice and a lot of sugar. Read the label.

Eating All-day events

All-day events like track meets or other sports tournaments where an athlete is expected to perform more than once, minutes to hours apart, present special problems. Make the most of a bad situation and remember that the basic pregame meal guidelines still apply.

You may have to eat several "mini" pregame meals over the day. Each meal should be small (under 300 calories) and low in sugar and fat. Even though schedules can be hectic, try to avoid eating within one hour of event time.

Sometimes, it's impossible to purchase suitable foods at the event. Many times, foods and drinks that are available at the refreshment stand (such as hot dogs, candy bars, and caffeinated drinks) are items that you shouldn't eat before performing. In these situations, you must plan ahead. For example, you can bring appropriate foods to the meet. Foods that spoil should be kept in coolers with ice to keep them cold.

Above all, drink plenty of fluids. Dehydration can be a very real danger at all-day events.

No Time ?

Plan ahead to have your favorite, quick, pregame foods on hand during the season. If possible, eat at least three hours before you compete.

If you only have time for a quick trip to the store, consider these possibilities:

- Oranges, bananas, pears, peaches, plums
- Juices
- Mozzarella string cheese
- Yogurt (low-fat)
- Single-portion cans of fruit
- Breadsticks/snacksticks
- Bread with jelly
- Cottage cheese (low-fat)
- Milk (low-fat or skim)

Ask your coach, food service director, or home economics teacher for refrigerator space if you need a pregame meal/snack right after school, between classes, or during a free period. A refrigerator and/or microwave would be a good booster club project.

Ask for nutritious foods in school vending machines: yogurt, fruit juices, and so on.

Bring a thermos of soup or a casserole from home.

Remember: Eat foods you like and that agree with you for pregame meals. You are an individual with your own tolerances for foods. Choosing foods you like may give you a psychological edge.

Energy Levels

Keeping your energy levels up for peak performance isn't easy. It doesn't just happen. High energy levels are the result of good eating and exercise habits. If you don't pay attention to either of these factors, your performance can suffer. Keeping Energy Levels Up will help you plan a diet for a winning performance.

One of the least-recognized nutrition problems of the young athlete is simply not eating enough. Extracurricular activities may make life so busy that you simply don't take the time to eat. After-school practice sessions may be so exhausting that you feel too tired to eat. But you must take the time to eat the right foods. Don't let fourth-quarter fatigue caused by poor eating hurt your performance.

Another problem of the young athlete is not eating the right kinds of foods—particularly foods high in starch. Eating a balanced diet that has plenty of starch keeps muscle energy up. Many young athletes eat more foods high in protein instead, and that's a mistake. A normal diet contains enough protein to support the added muscle growth and development of a young athlete.

Food Energy Needs Increase

Participating in sports can drastically increase your food energy needs. Increased physical activity calls for more food calories. Also, when you train, you increase muscle tissue relative to fat tissue, and muscle tissue requires more calories than fat tissue. Going out for sports can easily increase the daily calorie needs of a teen athlete by 2,000 or more. A teenage boy out for a sport like football or basketball may consume 5,000 or more calories daily.

The amount of food you need depends on your age, sex, weight, and activity level. A larger athlete requires more calories that a smaller one because more energy is needed to move more mass over the same distance. You usually burn more calories in a practice session than in actual competition because more total work is usually done during practice. However, the rate at which calories are burned for short periods of time may be greater from short bursts of intense activity during competition. Activity levels vary among sports as well as with the position played in a sport.

Obviously, it takes more energy to play basketball that baseball, and more energy to run 1,600 meters than the 100 meter dash.

If an athlete who is in shape loses body weight during a competitive season, it's a good indication that he or she isn't eating enough energy-providing food. Young athletes should be weighed once a week throughout the season to guard against unhealthy weight loss caused by inadequate food intake.

Food Strategy

All young athletes need to base their diets on a variety of nutritious foods. The Food Guide Pyramid is an excellent guide for young athletes to use because it

- helps you to select a variety of nutritious foods,
- emphasizes the starchy foods like breads, cereals, pastas, and vegetables you need to build glycogen stores,
- guides your selection of a lower fat diet, and
- offers you a variety of foods within each food group so that meals can be built around the foods you like.

Because of their rapid growth and development and higher levels of physical activity, many teen-athletes should eat the higher levels of servings recommended from each food group—especially from the bread, cereal, rice, and pasta group and the vegetable group. A 180-pound tight end could easily eat eleven servings of breads/cereals and five servings of vegetables daily. This athlete may even need more than the maximum servings recommended. Eating the maximum number of servings recommended from all five food groups provides about 3,000 calories. That's why large male athletes involved in a vigorous sport like football or soccer will have to eat more than the upper end of the recommended serving levels.

In no instance should you eat less than the minimum servings for any food group. You need the minimum servings to supply a base level of essential nutrients and calories required for good health. Consuming the minimum servings listed in the Food Guide Pyramid will supply about 1,600 calories, which is the minimum a teen girl should take in. Teen boys need at least 2,000 calories a day and thus need more than the minimums given.

Emphasize Starchy Food

Athletes need plenty of starchy foods because, along with proper training, these foods cause muscle and liver cells to store glycogen. Glycogen is a vital energy source for most sports. When muscle cells run out of glycogen, muscle fatigue sets in and performance suffers. Along with a proper exercise program, eating a normal, varied diet from the Food Guide Pyramid with emphasis on starchy foods will result in enough stored glycogen to carry you through 90 minutes of vigorous activity. And that's enough for most high-school activities.

Unfortunately, many girl athletes think of starchy foods as "fattening" and cut out breads, cereals, and starchy vegetables. The results are predictable: low glycogen, low energy, and poor performance. The girl athlete who wants top performance must eat starchy food so that she goes into an event with glycogen reserves. Starchy foods are not fattening in themselves. Eating more than you need of any food puts on pounds. The girl athlete who is training properly shouldn't worry about extra weight from starchy foods.

Teenage girls often have an incorrect perception of body image. Pounds that are added as a result of normal growth and development should not be confused with obesity. The percentage body fat should be monitored along with body weight. Most experts think that a teenage girl's body fat should not go below 12 to 14 percent.

Dried beans and peas contain some starch, and they can be used as a meat alternative because they contain ample protein. However, they can cause gas. Do not eat them for a pregame or prepractice meal unless you tolerate them well.

Energy packed meals

Some examples of high-starched meals that will help build and maintain adequate muscle glycogen are listed below. Pick the meals you like to eat, or make up your own meal that follows the same pattern as the Food Guide Pyramid recommendations. How much you eat depends on many factors: your age, sex, body size, and amount of physical activity. For example, a large male football player may eat at least two cups of chicken and noodles (Main Meal #1). On the other hand, a small female sprinter may eat only one cup.

If you eat generous amounts of the main dishes listed below, these meals supply over 1,000 calories and at least one-third of the recommended daily allowances (RDA) of most nutrients for teens. If you eat one serving of each food, the meals supply 55% to 62% of the energy as carbohydrate, 14% to 17% of the energy as protein, and 22% to 30% of the energy as fat.

Main Meal #1
Chicken and noodles/gravy
Whole wheat bread/jelly
Candied sweet potato
Fresh or cooked broccoli
Lowfat milk*
Orange juice
Main Meal #2
Hamburger/bun
Boston baked beans
Pear halves/lettuce
Cantaloupe
Lowfat milk*
Grape juice

Main Meal #3
Baked or broiled pork chop
Baked sweet potato
Lettuce and tomato salad/dressing
Banana
Whole wheat bread/jelly
Lowfat Milk*
Pineapple juice
Main Meal #4
Spaghetti and meatballs/Parmesan cheese
Italian bread/margarine
Carrot sticks
Peach halves/lettuce
Lowfat milk*
Apple juice
Main Meal #5
Macaroni and cheese
Cooked green beans
Fruit salad
Whole wheat bread/jelly/peanut butter
Lowfat milk*
Orange juice
Main Meal #6
Roast beef/stewed tomatoes
Baked potato/margarine
Whole wheat bread/jelly
Fresh fruit of choice
Lowfat milk*
Cranberry juice
*2 percent, 1 percent, and skim milk are all considered low fat.

Success Strategies before the game

The glycogen stores you have available right before an event are the result of how you've eaten and exercised for the past several days. Glycogen stores in the body are increased by rest or light levels of exercise and high levels of carbohydrates (particularly starch) in the diet. Glycogen stores in the body are lowered by high levels of exercise and low levels of starch in the diet. Once glycogen stores are exhausted, it takes at least two days to fully restore them. Although the pregame meal can stabilize blood sugar levels and provide some energy, don't look to the pregame meal to provide the bulk of your energy for the game.

You should eat a nutritious, varied diet containing plenty of starchy foods every day. Give starches particular emphasis two days before the event. Also, cut back on workouts a day or two before the event to increase glycogen stores. Most high-school coaches hold lighter workouts the day before a game. This gives glycogen levels a chance to build up.

Here are some tips to help you keep your glycogen reserves up—particularly for the big game.

- Start each day with a good breakfast. Cold cereal, milk, toast, fruit, and/or fruit juice make an easy-to-fix, quick meal that provides plenty of starch.
- Select meals that contain foods from all five food groups. Our bodies use nutrients more efficiently when they are consumed together.
- Use snacks as another opportunity to power up with starch—and don't forget that snack at bedtime. Cold cereal with milk serves as a quick snack at any time. It can be more than the "breakfast" of champions! And you don't have to stop at one bowlful.
- Give starchy foods particular emphasis the days right before the event by building the main meal around a high-starch entree like spaghetti and meatballs. Make sure the other food groups are also represented.
- Decrease physical activity the day before and the day of the event. Practices directed by your coach are enough. The day before or the day of the event is not the time to organize a pickup game with your friends. Rest up!
- Drink plenty of fluids—even at mealtimes—to guard against dehydration.

Eating strategies after the game

After the game or practice session, much of the glycogen in your muscle and liver tissue has been used up, and synthesis, or creation, of new muscle protein slows. To promote glycogen recovery, consume nutritious foods and drinks that are high in carbohydrates. When you eat the right foods, your body can replace lost glycogen rapidly, and normal synthesis of new proteins can resume.

Whole foods like cereals, breads, and pastas with a glass of milk are better for total recovery than pure carbohydrate supplements. A mix of whole foods contains proteins, minerals, and vitamins in addition to carbohydrates. You need these other nutrients along with high levels of carbohydrates for a complete, rapid recovery.

To insure that you get enough carbohydrates, take in one gram of carbohydrates for each kilogram (2.2 pounds) of body weight. For example, a 110 pound athlete should consume about 50 grams of carbohydrates for maximum glycogen replacement after an event. A 156-pound athlete would need about 70 grams of carbohydrates. One ounce of breakfast cereal contains about 20 grams of carbohydrates, and one slice of bread has about 12 grams. Remember, whole foods, such as breads and cereals, when eaten with beverages like milk promote more rapid recovery than pure carbohydrates alone.

To assist in total, rapid recovery, you should consume nutritious foods and drinks as soon as you can tolerate them after an event or workout. Ideally, you should eat food within two hours afterward. However, if you can't tolerate eating that soon, choose what's comfortable for you.

Remember to drink plenty of fluids, even if you aren't thirsty. Keep your fluid levels up!

Quick Energy Foods

Young athletes often have questions about foods high in fat and sugar, such as candy, pop, and desserts. These foods are called "empty calorie" foods because they're usually high in calories but contain few nutrients. Don't eat many of these foods. Get your energy from foods that supply ample proteins, vitamins, and minerals as well as calories.

Many athletes mistakenly believe that high-sugar foods will give them quick energy before a game or an event. High-sugar foods, such as candy or honey, should be avoided before a game or an event. Sweets can cause rapid swings in blood sugar, make you feel tired, and decrease performance.

Loading Carbohydrates

Should young athletes follow strict carbohydrate-loading routines often used by adult athletes who are involved in endurance events, such as marathon running or bicycling? Definitely not!

True carbohydrate loading is a rigid exercise and diet plan that adult athletes follow for the week right before the big event. During the first half of the week, glycogen stores are drained by exhaustive exercise and by a diet very low in starch. The athlete then gets a rebound effect during the second half of the week by eating a diet very high in starch and not exercising at all.

Such strict routines that drastically increase glycogen reserves are necessary only for marathon-type activities. These very high levels of glycogen are not needed for high-school sporting events. In fact, true carbohydrate loading can severely stress the body and cause heart and kidney problems. A high-school athlete should eat plenty of starch every day and not make drastic dietary swings from low to high levels of starch.

Fluid Levels

Water is a basic necessity for all life. Without it, life can't exist. Even when water is limited, living organisms suffer. You are no exception. For young athletes like yourself, not enough water means you can't do your best. It can even cause serious health problems.

Our blood circulates like an ocean within us. The water in blood helps carry nutrients and energy to our body cells. It also carries waste products away from our cells for excretion from our body. Water helps regulate our body temperature, too—an important factor for all of us.

As a young athlete, you have a special need for water. When you participate in a sport like track or volleyball, you burn a lot of food energy (called calories). Some of that unleashed energy powers muscles. But some of that energy is released as heat. Water keeps you from overheating. Sweating and evaporation from the skin cools you down. However, water is lost in the cooling process. That can be dangerous if the water is not replenished. If you run low on water, your body can overheat, like a car that is low on cooling fluid. Losing just two percent of the body's water can hurt performance. A five percent loss can cause heat exhaustion. A seven percent to ten percent loss can result in heat stroke and death. Dehydration can kill.

Young athletes have a lot of growing to do. New muscle tissue must be made. Bones need to grow rapidly. And with all of the physical activity, some tissues need to be repaired. All of this metabolic activity requires an abundance of nutrients and energy carried to body tissues and waste products carried away. Water allows all of this to happen. Water is vital for your body's growth, repair, and physical activity.

Thirst is your body's signal that you need to drink water. By the time you feel thirsty, you may have already lost one percent to two percent of your water—and that's enough to hurt performance. But just drinking enough to satisfy your thirst may not supply your body's needs. If you drink only enough to satisfy your thirst, your body may take up to 24 hours to fully rehydrate its cells and regain maximum performance.

When you participate in a sporting event or practice session, follow these guidelines:

- Don't wait until you are thirsty before drinking water.
- Drink more than enough to satisfy your thirst.
- Drink more than you think you need before an event or practice to make sure you are fully rehydrated.

There is an old misconception that is dying hard. It is similar to the hard-line "no pain: no gain" training philosophy that we now know is also false.

Many coaches and athletes once believed that restricting water during a competition or practice session toughened an athlete—that somehow athletes needed less water. Unfortunately, some people still follow this practice that lowers performance and is downright dangerous. Without enough water to cool itself, the body can overheat to dangerous levels.

Conditioned athletes need more water—not less. The conditioned athlete is able to store and burn more energy in a shorter time. That means your body releases more heat, requires more cooling, loses more water, and needs more water to replenish its stores. Also, you may have increased your sweating response, which means you lose even more water. As an in-shape athlete, you need more water than other people.

When you feel exhausted and hot during a workout or game, drinking large amounts of water very rapidly may cause discomfort or stomach cramps. But that is not a good reason to restrict water. Drinking moderate amounts at frequent intervals is the best strategy during competition or practice. About one cup (six to eight ounces) of cool water every 15 to 20 minutes during an activity is about right for most athletes. Some athletes can drink a bit more than this at each interval. Cool water (40 to 50 degrees Fahrenheit) is best. Cool water helps absorb body heat. And it empties from the stomach into the intestine at a fast rate, which allows it to be absorbed rapidly into the body.

Most of the weight you lose during an event or training session is water lost through sweat. Of course, you lose some weight when your body burns materials for energy. For example, the glycogen stored in liver and muscle cells is used for energy, which results in some weight loss. Some fat and protein is burned for energy, too, and that results in additional weight loss. However, most of the weight you lose during strenuous physical activity is water lost through perspiration.

Some coaches and trainers weigh athletes before a contest or workout and then again after the activity is over. Before the athletes leave the facility, they are encouraged to drink water until they are within one pound of their pre-session weight. Two eight-ounce cups of water are consumed for each pound lost. This practice—weighing in, weighing out, and drinking the difference—is an excellent way of guarding against dehydration. You can do this on your own even if your coach doesn't require it.

Dehydration is not a way to make weight

At one time, wrestlers purposely dehydrated to lose weight rapidly and make weight categories. Fortunately, this practice is decreasing, but it still occurs.

Wrestlers dehydrated in many ways. Some exercised in hot rooms, often while wearing rubber suits in an attempt to sweat off water. Others simply did not drink any fluids or eat foods high in water. Still others lost water by spitting in a cup all day. And some took diuretics (water pills) to increase urine output.

Unfortunately, a few wrestlers used a combination of these methods to reduce body water, lose weight, and make weight categories. None of these practices is recommended. Using them in combination is especially dangerous.

Dehydration poses both short- and long-term dangers to your health. In the short-term, your body's cooling system can't work properly and you can overheat, suffer heatstroke, and possibly die. Long-term, repeated episodes of dehydration can be damaging to your kidneys.

The most common outcomes of dehydration are poor endurance and poor performance. Some athletes mistakenly believe that after purposely dehydrating their bodies, they can rapidly rehydrate and almost immeditaley regain optimum performance. While drinking plenty of fluids is the right thing to do after becoming dehydrated, it may take many hours before your body completeley rehydrates and you can perform your best.

Some drinks that have caffeine, such as colas and iced tea, are advertised as thirst quenchers. Do not use caffeine-containing beverages as fluid rehydration drinks shortly before, during, and after a practice or competition. Caffeine acts as a diuretic. It increases urine output and can promote dehydration.

Necessity of sports drinks

Your biggest concern is getting enough water—pure, cool water. Even the salt you lose while sweating can be easily replaced by adding salt to foods.

Plain, cool water is the fluid of choice when the actual exercise does not last longer than 60 to 90 minutes. And that includes most situations, even a tough practice session, a hard-fought football game, or a track meet. You don't need an energy source in the fluid you drink to rehydrate. During these normal situations, if you have been eating and training properly, you should have enough energy stored as liver and muscle glycogen to power you through.

However, in some situations where the exercise is unusually long or several games occur in a short period of time, sport drinks containing carbohydrates and electrolytes may offer you an advantage. During these situations, you may run low on energy and electrolytes. For example, if you are a long-distance cyclist, you should consider using a sport drink. If you must compete in a tournament that has more than one game a day or several games in just a few days, you could benefit from a sport drink that supplements your energy and electrolyte supply.

There are many different commercial sport drinks available. They contain varying kinds and amounts of carbohydrates and electrolytes. For example, GATORADE® Thirst Quencher is a glucose electrolyte solution of about six percent carbohydrate concentration. Exceed® is a glucose polymer solution of about seven percent carbohydrate concentration. If you use a sport drink, pick one that has less than eight percent total solids (carbohydrates, electrolytes). More concentrated solutions can delay fluid absorption. They must be diluted with plain water before you use them as a fluid replacement drink. Also, avoid sport drinks that contain fructose as the only source of carbohydrate. Fructose may delay gastric emptying of fluid and cause upset stomach. And fructose must first be converted to glucose before it can be used for energy. This conversion means you can't use fructose as an energy source as quickly as other carbohydrates.

Fruit juices like orange juice should also be diluted if you're using them as a fluid replacement drink before, during, or after an event or practice session. Fruit juices vary from 10% to 17% carbohydrate concentration. Dilute them with an equal amount of pure water before you use them as fluid replacement. Of course, when you drink juices at other times, such as with a meal or snack, you don't have to dilute them.

Take every opportunity to drink water and other appropriate fluids. Drink fluids every day, even when you are not thirsty. That means drinking at mealtime—and snacktime, too! As a competition or practice approaches, follow these guidelines:

- Drink plenty of appropriate fluids the 24 hours before an event. Give your body every opportunity to become fully rehydrated.
- If you eat a pregame meal three or more hours before an event, make sure that ample fluids are included—at least two cups (16 ounces).
- About 15 to 30 minutes before the start of competition or practice, drink a cup or more of fluids. This will help ensure that your tissues are fully rehydrated at the start.
- During the activity, drink six to eight ounces of fluids every 15 to 20 minutes. Drinking moderate amounts frequently is the best way to keep fluid levels up. If you drink too much too quickly, you may develop stomach cramps and other discomfort.
- Drink plenty of fluids after the activity. If you weigh in before and after activities, drink two cups (16 ounces) for every pound lost until you are within a pound of your pre-activity weight.
- Remember to drink fluids before you get thirsty. If you wait until you're thirsty, your body may have already lost enough water to hurt your performance.

Getting it all down means you can perform at your best levels. Your endurance will be long lasting and you won't become as tired. You will have that extra edge when you need it most—whether it's the last few minutes of the contest or the last 10 meters before the finish line.

Remember to power up with good food every day so you can take full advantage of a well-hydrated body.

CHAPTER 4

HEALING THROUGH FOOD

Leafy Green Vegetables and Fruits for Antioxidants-
Leafy green vegetables provide antioxidants that build the immune system to fight off illness and dis-ease. Antioxidants are protection from harmful free radicals that can damage and reduce healthy cells and promote the cell aging process.

Antioxidants Free/ radicals cause irreversible damage (oxidation) to cells like rust on a pipe. They form and grow on the damage done in your body from smoking, exhaust fumes, radiation, excessive sunlight, certain drugs, intensive exercise without proper nutrition, stress and abnormal metabolism. As free radicals build they damage your healthy cells, ultimately this speeds the cell aging process because they eave your body vulnerable to advanced aging, cancer, cardiovascular disease and degenerative diseases like arthritis. Your body has a natural antioxidant mechanism that protects you from most cell damage. Fruits and leafy green vegetables have substances in them that act as antioxidants. Antioxidants are available as supplements such as Vitamins C and E, Selenium, Phytonutrients including beta-Carotene, lycopine and lutein free radicals. Soybeans are Natural Estrogen - Soybeans contain isoflavinoids that are actually weak estrogen. These compounds ease menopausal symptoms and reduce the risk of uterine colon and breast cancers. It also lowers LDL level cholesterol. You can get soybeans in a Soya protein powder. This powder mix is filled with amino acids that aide in memory retention, weight loss and increases muscle. Pregnant women especially should consult with their physician before taking soy products.

Vitamin Functions -

Cancer Prevention: Last year, the American Institute for Cancer Research launched a new educational program called "The New American Plate," which calls for Americans to shift the proportions on their plates for lower weight and better health. By emphasizing how healthy proportions will look on the plate ("two-thirds or more vegetables, fruits, whole grains and beans; one-third or less animal protein") and offering recipes that emphasize the flavors, colors and textures of plant foods, the New American Plate has helped thousands of people consume a more varied and healthy diet.

Lutein: Spinach, avocado and other yellow or leafy green vegetables contain lutein which concentrates in the retina and the lens where it reduces the risk for cataracts and macular degeneration, the leading preventable cause of blindness in America, which affects 13 million people. Surprisingly, he said, lutein also slows prostate cancer cell growth. And when it is combined with lycopine, lutein demonstrates independent and additive preventive effects on prostate cancer cell growth.

Essential fatty acids (EFA's) are "good" fats necessary for producing new cell membranes. What scientists are discovering about EFA's is especially encouraging relative to the eyes. We already know that omega-3 and omega-6 fatty acids, for example, have a wonderful track record for enhancing the health of the heart and balancing water in the body. Recently, researchers have learned that these fatty acids also help maintain the delicate fluid balance in the eyes.

St John's Wort is nicknamed herbal Prozac. This herb is thought to act in the same way as some antidepressants by enhancing the effect of the neurotransmitter, serotonin, in the brain. It has a long history of use. One of the rare side-effects of St John's Wort is an increase in sensitivity to light. This may also explain why it is effective for treating SAD (Seasonal Affective Disorder) related depression in the winter.

Benefits of Uncooked Natural Foods: Avoiding cooking prevents the hazards of the microwave, of burns, of fires, of enzyme destruction, of carcinogens created by heat, the cost of cooking, the time of cooking and of cleanup, carcinogens in metal cookware such as aluminum, etc.

Low Acid Foods - Many diseases come from over acidification of the body. Meat, eggs, fish, nicotine, coffee have high acid contents. Fruits, even citrus fruits, are excellent for potassium which offsets sodium and acidification. Fruits with average levels of potassium include apricots, peaches, bananas, raisins (1/2 cup), prunes, cantaloupe, figs, dates, watermelon, and juices such as orange, grapefruit, tangerine and prunes. Fruits in general are alkaline and therefore reverse acidification.. Even citrus has a biochemical change in the body.

Kidney stones are caused by excess calcium (in animal products), excess oxalic acid (from the cooking of some vegetables, and other factors. The thin green layer between potato's brown skin and white interior when cooked causes oxalic acid, e.g. Fruitarians in general have the fewest kidney stones. If you like fried potatoes it is better to cook them in olive oil and to peel them to avoid the oxalates

Fruit has the most natural fiber for good intestinal function, those who eat lots of fruit have the least intestinal cancer, constipation, appendicitis, hemorrhoids, peritonitis; etc. Citrus fruit becomes alkaline in processing. Fruit is the least acid of all foods and therefore the food which is best for long life.

The basic elements of the Lifestyle diet

1. Air, Do breathing exercises, and breathe fresh air from nature.
2. Water: Flushes interior and outside of body. Drink bottles of organic water a day to flush out impurities, to flatten and clear out food in the stomach, to clean the skin, etc.
3. Sun: The rays of the sun are good for your pineal glands, and decreases depression, sunlight aids in uplifting the mind body and spirit
4. Food: Natural food that is fresh raw fruits and vegetables, reduce carbohydrates, vegan or vegetarian or reduce meat in the diet;
5. Movement, Exercise
6. Cleansing the internal organs through water, herbal therapies and occasional
7. Organic minerals, comprised of the body elements and earth elements

Almonds contain a high percentage of essential amino compounds and are rich in protein. Although the percentage of fat is high, it's an unsaturated oil that is readily digested and assimilated. Almonds have an alkaline effect in the body, the most complete alkaline of any other nut. They are helpful in the treatment of heartburn and peptic ulcers. It's the oil and protein in the nut, and their interaction with the gastric juices/acids.that promotes this beneficial effect.

Almonds are also credited as a cure for cancer. Dr. Harold Manna in his book "The Death of Cancer" explains how amygdaline destroys cancer cells. Amygdaline is present in the sweet almond however the bitter almond contains a ferment, emulsion which is missing from the sweet variety (found in apricot/peach pits) The effective agent in amygdaline appears to be a vitamin designated as B-17. As well, the almond has a decent amount Cyanic Acid content (cyanide) within. Unlike regular healthy cells,cancer cells function without oxidative mechanisms and soak up the Cyanic Acid which destroys cancer cells.

Remedies in Foods

Natural Nutrition

Soy protein is now recognized as the only complete protein from a plant source. That means soy protein contains all of the essential amino acids that you must get from food. These amino acids are present in just the right balance to meet your body's need for protein. More good news - soy protein is equal in protein quality to animal proteins such as meat, milk, and egg proteins.

Scientific Research on Soy Protein

Here's some recent clinical and demonstrative research on how soy protein has definite and positive benefits in your performance and health diets.

Cardiovascular disease (CVD) refers to diseases and conditions that affect your heart and arteries, including heart attack, stroke and high blood pressure. Although CVD is a major cause of death in the United States and most developed countries, not all populations have the same degree of risk.

Compare death rates from CVD in the United States and Japan, for example, and you'll see startling differences. CVD death rates for both men and women are more than twice as high in the United States than in Japan. The second area of interest involves soy and the effect it could have on the prevalence of several common chronic diseases. These include heart disease and some specific cancers, among others.

Epidemiology also reveals significant differences between East and West in death rates from certain cancers. Breast cancer in women and prostate cancer in men are the most common cancers and second leading causes of cancer death in Americans. Comparisons of death rates from these cancers in the United States and Japan show that, here again, the Japanese have a clear health advantage.

Compared with the Japanese, death rates for breast cancer are more than 2 ½ times higher in American women and death rates for prostate cancer are more than three times higher in American men.

Although there are many differences between East and West, a great deal of interest focused on diet, and specifically soy protein consumption.

On average, Americans consume only 1-3 grams of soy protein a day. The average soy protein intake in Asia, on the other hand, ranges from about 10 grams a day in China to 30-50 grams a day in Japan and Taiwan.3 As a rule, Asians average consuming 20-50 times more soyfoods than Americans.

However, when Asians migrate to the West, their diets change over time. In one survey, the soyfood intake of Chinese people living in China was 10 - 15 times higher than that of Chinese people in California and Hawaii.

They found that, compared with Caucasians, breast cancer risk was about 50% lower in women born in Asia and 25% lower in American-born Asians.6 Other researchers have noted that as Japanese men move from Japan to parts of the world where prostate cancer is more common, their incidence increases.

Health Tips

Eat some foods high in potassium and calcium every day.

The chemical reactions inside all our cells are very sensitive to the balance of acid and alkali. This balance is maintained by ions of calcium, potassium, sodium, chloride, phosphate and hydrogencarbonate.

If we eat excess protein or acid foods, calcium and potassium ions get used up in order to neutralise the acid. Dr Hay and modern science advocate the same two approaches. Don't eat too much protein and do eat high potassium foods every day. Dr Hay also advocates restricting the intake of acid foods such as rhubarb and vinegar, but modern food chemistry demonstrates that a touch of vinegar in cooking a protein meal will help preserve many of the vitamins such as thiamin, riboflavin, folate and vitamin C.

Women - require only one starch meal each day unless you are active and need the extra energy.

Men - need extra energy and may require two starch meals a day.

On average women have a more efficient metabolism than men. If you have a very low fat diet, you will need to eat more starch than you can comfortably eat in one sitting. If you have a physically active life, two starch meals a day may give you all the energy that you need.

Non-starchy vegetables may not provide you with vast amounts of energy, but they do provide important essential vitamins, minerals and trace elements. Eat a wide variety and use them to fill up your plate at any meal. Use fresh or frozen vegetables and cook by steaming or microwaving for the best nutritional value.

There is no one food that has all the ingredients we need. If we eat a wide variety, we ensure that we get sufficient of all the vitamins and minerals that our bodies require. There is some evidence that eating a little of a lot of different foods greatly reduces the chances of developing food allergies. This applies particularly to the main starch foods so don't eat wheat and potatoes all the time.

"Which Way to Health" recommends that you eat as much as you like of fruit and vegetables. Your target should be five portions a day. They're full of vitamins and fibre, but low in calories. Don't worry too much about pesticides in or on fruit: for most of us, heart disease is a much bigger risk. If you are worried, buy organic, or grow your own.

In the UK the highest incidence of heart disease occurs in the people who eat the least fruit and vegetables. The more fruit and vegetables you eat, the less likely you are to develop cancer of the lung, stomach, mouth, cervix, colon or rectum.

Fresh fruit contain far more vitamins than cooked fruit. They make ideal snacks between meals and are superb for that 'feel good' factor.

Some fruits, like bananas, dates and plantains are starchy. Others, like citrus fruit, are acid. Most can be eaten with any protein meal.

Use olive oil if you need extra oil for cooking or dressings

Olive oil is an easily digested, mono-unsaturated oil and is a good source of vitamin E. Extra virgin cold pressed oil is best. It is the basic oil of the healthy Mediterranean lifestyle. Cretans in particular have the second lowest rate of heart disease in the world.

Butter or margarine? Should you eat saturated fats or polyunsaturated fats? Margarines are highly processed and refined foods. If you keep your fat intake low, you can allow yourself butter and cream (1oz / 25g of each per day) Both these are pure, natural foods.

You can eat butter and cream in moderation

Butter is an excellent source of vitamin E and is pure dairy fat. Single cream is 20% fat and is a good source of vitamins A, E and D.

A certain amount of fat is essential in our diet. Provided that your overall intake of fat is kept low, butter and cream will enhance your lifestyle and help you maintain your health.

Don't smother starch meals in fat.

A healthy starch meal can easily be overloaded with an unhealthy fatty sauce. A baked potato with a small lump of butter or potato chips dipped in olive oil and drained before roasting in the oven make excellent meals, but if the potato is soaked in fat, you will suffer all the risks of a high fat diet.

Sugar is absorbed too quickly into the blood stream. It results in swings in blood sugar level that put a strain on all the regulation systems in the body. High blood sugar levels can increase damage in all the tissues that the blood bathes.

Sugar adds nothing useful to the diet. You get a much more useful supply of energy from eating starchy foods.

Black treacle, molasses and honey contain useful minerals and vitamins. Use these in moderation.

Salt, or sodium chloride, is essential in very small amounts in our diet, but it is easy to eat far too much. The surplus salt has to be excreted by the kidneys. This makes the kidneys work harder and increases the risk of kidney failure.

Salt can also prevent uptake of calcium and lead to poor bone development in children.

Cholesterol is an essential compound, most of which is manufactured in our livers, and circulated throughout our bodies. High-cholesterol foods such as shell-fish and eggs are now thought to have little effect on blood cholesterol levels. Low cholesterol levels can result in severe depression.

You can slash your risk of heart disease still further by eating two portions of oily fish, such as herring or mackerel each week. Blood pressure and inflammation can be reduced and controlled by eating fish oils that contain omega-3 fatty acids. The best sources of these are mackerel, sardines, salmon, pilchards and herring. But note; you can overdose on fish oil supplements - vitamins A & D are toxic in high amounts.

Eating excessive amounts of bran can prevent your body absorbing essential calcium, iron, zinc and copper. Wheat fibre can be rough and irritating to the human digestive system. If you eat whole grain cereals and plenty of fresh fruit and vegetables, you don't need to add extra fibre to your diet.

Another New Scientist report states that "New research from Britain and the US, as well as Japan, provides strong evidence that women can substantially reduce the risk of breast cancer by consuming soya bean products, such as soya milk, or tofu."

A diet high in soya protein can alter women's hormones in a way that mimics the anti cancer drug tamoxifen. Eating soya products can lower the risk of both prostate and colon cancers." "Most natural high fibre foods, such as whole wheat, oats, barley, rye, sesame and flax seeds may have a similar effect.

- Borage seed oil (starflower oil) is high in Gamma Linolenic Acid. Its anti inflammatory properties helps reduce swelling and tenderness of joints in rheumatoid arthritis. It has higher levels of this acid than evening primrose oil.
- Cranberry juice can help protect against all types of urinary infections according to researchers at Boston USA.
- Garlic has strong antibiotic properties.
- Don't go on a calorie reduced diet to slim without taking plenty of exercise. Without the exercise you lose muscle, not fat. You'll end up weak and fat!
- Red wine in moderation is good for older people only! A lot still damages your liver. For younger people the risks of developing liver cancer outweigh the health benefits of a glass of wine.
- Suffer from mouth ulcers? You may be short of B vitamins, particularly thiamine, riboflavin and B6.
- Women who suffer prolonged or heavy periods are likely to develop an iron deficiency.
- Women who have premenstrual syndrome may lack vitamins B and C.
- Vegetarians may develop iron deficiency.
- Convenience foods are often low in vitamin B and magnesium.
- If you don't eat fresh fruit and vegetables every day you may lack vitamin C, magnesium and potassium.
- Heavy smokers need a much higher intake of vitamin C for good health.
- Older people need to increase their intake of vitamin B, calcium, potassium and iron.

- Are you tired all the time? Researchers at Addenbrooke's Hospital in Cambridge think low levels of folic acid might be part of the cause.

Exercise

It does not matter what age you are. You need exercise to stay fit and healthy.

You are aiming at a minimum of three sessions of thirty minutes vigorous exercise each week. A better target is a thirty minute session every day. If you try to do too much too quickly you risk damage to joints and muscles and will end up stiff and sore.

If you are not fit now, you must start slowly and build yourself up. Time yourself with an alarm clock. Start with just one minute of exercise on the first day, two minutes on the second day, three minutes on the third. Continue adding just one minute to the exercise period each day, until at the end of 30 days you will have painlessly achieved your target - which you must now maintain every day!

It is best to select several different types of exercise that you really enjoy, and can keep going. The exercise should leave you feeling good, looking forward to the next session. The exercise should also develop stamina, strength and suppleness. Swimming hard is one of the few exercises that develops all three at the same time.

Vigorous exercise should leave you puffed, hot and sweaty! But if you feel muscle pain, stop. If you feel dizzy, or break out in a cold sweat, or suffer pains in the chest, neck or upper left arm, stop, and if this happens again consult your doctor.

If you are very unfit it may be wise to check with a doctor before you start a new exercise programme, particularly if you are over 60. You should also check with your doctor if you have high blood pressure, heart disease, joint pains or diabetes.

It is not wise to exercise strongly within two hours of a meal, within one hour of drinking alcohol, or in very hot or very cold conditions. But gentle exercise helps digestion. During gentle exercise, the muscles of the abdomen gently massage the digestive system, encouraging it to mix and move the digesting food. Tight belts or corsets can restrict the digestive system and produce symptoms of indigestion.

Relaxation

Stress in excess is also the cause of a wide range of disorders, both mental and physical. The food combining diet seems to make us more resilient to excess stress, but we need to be aware of the symptoms, and take control of our own lives. Stress can result from any situation where we feel we are not confident, and in control. Such situations cannot always be avoided, but we can recognise the symptoms and take steps to reduce the level of stress that we experience.

Stress can result in difficulty in sleeping, or sleeping too much when we don't want to wake up and face the world. It can cause appetite problems, indigestion and stomach upsets, diahorrea and frequent urination. It can produce headaches, muscle tension, clenched jaws and grinding teeth. It can result in nervousness, mood swings, irritability and angry outbursts.

Identifying the sources of stress and recognising how they are effecting you is the first step to keeping stress under control. If possible stop for a few minutes and take several slow deep breaths before continuing, and ensure you get a good night's sleep.

- Eat a light starch meal early in the evening.
- Avoid drinking tea, coffee or alcohol after mid afternoon.
- Ensure you have enough exercise every day.
- Check that your bed is comfortable and your bedroom at a reasonable temperature.
- Don't watch exciting TV or video programmes - or the news - last thing at night.
- Keep a pad and pen by the bed and jot down any ideas you want to remember, don't try to solve your problems last thing at night.

A caterpillar on your cauliflower is a sign that both are safe to eat!

Wash all fruit and vegetables well and discard the outer layers where these may accumulate pesticides. The only way of being sure that your vegetables are free of pesticides is to grow them yourselves, but you will then discover how hard it is to produce the unblemished pest-free produce on the supermarket shelves without the aid of pesticides.

Pesticides are probably more harmful than no pesticides, because many are nerve poisons and can accumulate to dangerous levels in the body over many years. But for many people in the world the choice is to accept a low pesticide residue on their food, or starve to death as a host of pests decimate the worlds crops while they grow, or destroy crops while in storage.

Aluminium in the diet is best kept as low as possible because of potential harm to the brain and the nervous system. Aluminium pots and pans are safe to use, provided they are NOT cleaned until shiny!

Aluminium protects itself with a hard layer of dull grey oxide. This will prevent any aluminium dissolving in the food. Provided this layer is left intact, aluminium is safe to use. Always wash aluminium with a soft cloth and detergent. Never scour it clean. Any food that leaves the pan bright and shiny - such as rhubarb or vinegar - should not be cooked in aluminium pans.

Cooking food may destroy enzymes and the chemicals which plants produce in order to try to prevent them being palatable to animals. This may improve the flavour, texture and digestibility of the raw food.

Cooking foods in liquid and then throwing away the liquid is very wasteful of many nutrients, particularly the water soluble vitamins such as thiamin, riboflavin, niacin and vitamin C. There is almost never any need to discard cooking water if the right amount is used in the first place. Any surplus liquid should be used for soups and gravies, or even, as in China, served as a cold drink.

The most nutrients are lost at high temperatures and by prolonged cooking. Foods left to stand may also lose nutrients.

Microwave and infra-red cooking can improve the nutritional status of food by reducing the use of liquids and cooking times. They are a good way of reheating food, provided the food is heated right through.

Cooking protein and starches together results in destruction of the amino acid lysine, severely degrading the quality of the protein. Prolonged cooking of protein can also make it more difficult to digest.

Freezing is the best method of storing food, although the blanching of food can reduce the thiamin and vitamin C content - but this is less than the loss that takes place in vegetables in a box during transport to and from a shop. Frozen foods should be kept below -18 C (0 F) until required for use.

Food that is processed for storage in tins, cans or glass jars will lose nutrients such as thiamin, folate and vitamin C as a result of the heat treatment. Other nutrients may be lost if a glass jar of food is stored in daylight.

Sulphur dioxide which is used as a preservative completely destroys all thiamin but helps to preserve vitamin C.

Prolonged drying in bright sunshine also destroys many of the vitamins in the food. Dried foods should be stored in sealed containers to exclude both oxygen and light.

Fibre & Constipation

The muscles of the walls of the small and large intestine push and pinch the digesting food, mixing it with enzymes, bringing it into close contact with the villi which absorb the nutrients, and ensuring the undigested food remains pass easily through the system. These muscles require something to push against. If the food is always soft or semi liquid, these muscles lose their strength, pockets and bulges form in the intestine walls where debris accumulates and waste becomes difficult to eliminate.

Fibre gives bulk to the food in the system and ensures that these muscles maintain their strength and can control the movement of food. The fibre also ensures that no pockets of debris are left behind and the whole digestive system operates efficiently and is self cleansing.

The most useful fibre comes from several portions a day of fresh fruit and vegetables, and from whole grain cereals. Added fibre is not nearly as useful and wheat fibre is not a useful addition to the diet. Wheat fibre is too abrasive and can obstruct the absorption of minerals.

Small children should not be fed on high fibre foods other than fresh fruit and vegetables.

Avoidable foods

Rhubarb and cooked tomato were also reputed to be excessively acid.

Modern methods of food analysis and a much greater understanding of the process of digestion and absorption of food can help clarify the position.

Fruit acids should not be a problem, Fresh acid fruit are an essential part of a balanced and healthy diet. They should be eaten on their own or as part of a protein meal.

Vinegar is a weak solution of ethanoic acid and this is metabolised to carbon dioxide and water. The carbon dioxide is eliminated with exhaled air and places less of a burden on the digestive system than alcohol. Vinegar should be eaten with protein rather than with starch, as it will prevent the action of the starch enzymes in the mouth. The slight acidity will also preserve the vitamins in a protein meal. Lemon juice can be used in place of vinegar in most recipes.

Similarly, cooked tomato should not be a problem as part of a protein meal, and it will also help preserve the vitamin content of the meal.

Rhubarb contains oxalic acid. In early spring when the amount of oxalate in the stem is low, rhubarb can safely be eaten, but by the end of May, the concentration is starting to rise and rhubarb should be avoided. The oxalic acid also prevents the absorbtion of calcium from food and so should not be eaten on a regular basis. The leaves of rhubarb should never be eaten.

Far more dangerous to eat are foods made from mixtures of fat and sugar such as biscuits and cakes.

Fat and sugar mixtures are a double danger to our bodies. Because the ingredients are highly refined, we don't know when we have eaten enough. The refined fats are absorbed quickly into the bloodstream where they coat and clog blood vessels, and have to be stored quickly in fatty tissue. The sugar has equally serious effects on the body's mechanisms. Almost all medical opinions and government health guidelines now agree that sugar and fat mixtures make a major contribution to heart disease and cancer. Avoid them!

Chocolate is also a fat sugar mixture that includes traces of drugs that can cause cravings and addiction. The amount of chocolate in the diet should severely restricted.

Changing the Diet

Combining Food

Food Combining is designed to improve your quality of life. It is not a penance that you should endure. It will keep you alert and fit and following it should not make you anxious and worried.

Any move towards the Food Combining lifestyle will help you improve your health and fitness. It is not an all or nothing diet, and it doesn't have to be adopted in full all at once.

It's even better if you don't change too quickly! The digestive system needs time to adapt to the new improved regime and to new foods. But start by reducing your consumption of sugar / fat mixtures such as biscuits, cake and pastry, and replace them with fresh fruit.

Try not to eat until you are hungry, don't eat out of habit, and don't eat everything just because it is offered to you. Drink whenever you are thirsty, clean water is always the best way to quench a thirst.

The next step is to reduce your intake of concentrated protein - meat, fish, cheese, beans to just one meal a day.

Slowly increase the amount of exercise that you take. It need only be by a couple of minutes each day.

Food Combining is the easy way to plan an interesting, varied and healthy diet.

You don't need to count calories or measure portions. You will soon discover how much you want to eat.

Chose as wide a range of ingredients as are easily available and you will almost certainly get a balanced diet.

Fill up with the starchy items for breakfast and lunch, and with the vegetables and fruit for the main meal.

Sample Menu for Healthy Living :

Sunday	breakfast oatmeal porridge	lunch potato roast fresh fruit salad	main meal roast chicken with a selection of root and leaf vegetables (not potatoes) lemon cream
Monday	breakfast muesli	lunch hot garlic potatoes and salad banana	main Meal cheese pudding with a selection of vegetables
Tuesday	breakfast cornflakes with yogurt and sultanas	lunch bread, butter and salad	main meal poached fish with selection of vegetables(not potatoes), apple pudding
Wednesday	breakfast millet and date porridge	lunch pasta with a pesto sauce	main meal cottage pie fresh fruit
Thursday	breakfast polenta	lunch cashew nut pilaf fresh fruit	main meal turkey moussaka with selection of vegetables (not potatoes), dried fruit salad
Friday	breakfast toast and marmalade	lunch rice salad fresh fruit	main meal baked mackerel with a selection of vegetables (not potatoes), cheeses

Saturday	breakfast rice and sultanas	lunch baked potato	main meal Citrus and Almond turkey with a selection of vegetables (not potatoes) Lemon cream, cheeses
Sunday	breakfast yogurt and fresh fruit	lunch cauliflower and potato soup fresh fruit salad	main meal roast ham with a selection of root and leaf vegetables (not potatoes) apple pudding
Monday	breakfast muesli	lunch pasta with pesto salad dried fruit salad	main Meal sausages with a selection of vegetables
Tuesday	breakfast cornflakes with banana	lunch wholemeal pizza and salad	main meal blue cheese and walnut sauce with a selection of vegetables(not potatoes), fresh fruit
Wednesday	breakfast mixed grain bread, toasted	lunch persian style rice	main meal casserole of hearts, Greek salad fresh fruit
Thursday	breakfast muesli	lunch naan bread fresh fruit	main meal mutton or beef stew
Friday	breakfast toast and marmalade	lunch rice salad fresh fruit	main meal grilled herring with a selection of vegetables

Pressure Cooking

The speed and efficiency of the microwave oven has caused many people to leave their pressure cookers unused at the back of a cupboard. But there is still a place for this useful item in every kitchen, and there are many dishes which are best and quickest cooked in this way. Not only does the pressure cooker save fuel by cooking so quickly (a third of the time is a good general rule) but it also blends the flavours and tenderises meat in a way that the average microwave cannot match.

A pressure cooker is a large saucepan with a lid, which is usually very deep. (I would always buy the one with the deep lid rather than the shallow, as you can then pile up such foods as Christmas puddings and cook two or three at once, making a further saving on fuel.) The lid is sealed with a rubber gasket and there is a control vent in the top with a safety plug.

The cooker is designed to make use of the steam given off by foods as they cook, or by the water they are cooked in, by confining it so that there is a rise in pressure inside the cooker and a corresponding rise in temperature. The combination of increased pressure and higher temperature forces steam through the food and reduces the cooking time.

The pressure is controlled by small weights which are fitted on the lid - High pressure (15 lb) is suitable for general cooking purposes; Medium (10 lb) is used for pre-cooking fruits for jam; Low (5 lb) is best for cooking steamed puddings. Christmas puddings are especially good cooked in a pressure cooker. The appropriate pressure is always indicated in recipes. Timing starts from when the cooker reaches pressure after the weight is placed on the lid.

Pressure cookers are easy to use, but care must be taken when opening after cooking is finished. The cooker must always be cooled, either by allowing to cool gradually off the heat or by holding under cold running water, and the weight must not be removed until the cooker has stopped hissing. (My mother did this once when cooking beetroot, with the result that the newly-painted kitchen ceiling and walls were suddenly splattered with purple. More importantly, she could have been badly scalded.) Always follow the manufacturer's instructions.

The pressure cooker also has a trivet, which is used inside the cooker to keep foods out of the liquid necessary to produce steam. Vegetables, for instance, are not cooked in water but in steam, and only a small amount of water is needed.Other foods, like steamed puddings, might burn if allowed contact with the bottom of the cooker, so they too can be stood on the trivet.

Some pressure cookers have baskets or separators which can be fitted inside the cooker in order to cook several different foods at once. For instance, turnips may be laid on the trivet and the separators rested on top, two containing different vegetables and one with meat.

If you live over 2,000 feet above sea-level, the cooking must be calculated differently. Again, follow the manufacturer's instructions but in most cases the time will not be increased by more than one minute for every thousand feet and it may be recommended that you simply use a different weight.

Average times for foods cooked in the pressure cooker
Potatoes - 6 minutes
Carrots - 6 minutes
Meat stew - 20 minutes
Braised stuffed sheeps' hearts - 30 minutes
Fish - 4 minutes
Christmas pudding - 2lb pudding at 30 minutes steaming (without the weights) and 3 hours at 15lb pressure. If you have a cooker with a high lid, you can cook two puddings together at the same time.

Soups are wonderful made in the pressure cooker. In our house a chicken is never allowed to leave the house until every atom of goodness has been extracted by boiling it up in the pressure cooker. Bacon knuckles also produce a very good soup, with vegetables and lentils. The vegetables can be fresh or leftover and quantities can be varied according to taste or what you have.

Slow cookers are designed to cook at 92 degrees Celsius. They should reach this temperature on a high setting within thirty minutes, or longer on a slow setting.

Slow cooking can improve the eating qualities of tough joints of meat, but they are not suitable for beans as the temperature is too low to destroy toxins in the beans.

Food should never be left to keep warm in the slow cooker. It should either be served hot, or cooled and refrigerated. Some slow cookers have caused problems because they don't reach a high enough temperature.

Woks

These are ideal for heat sealing and fast cooking. Food should always be kept on the move to prevent overcooking.

Microwave Oven

These work well for small quantities of moist food. For larger quanitites they have no advantage over conventional cooking methods. Vegetables cooked in the microwave can retain higher levels of vitamins than boiled vegetables. Large items of foods can retain cold spots in the microwave and need to stand until the heat is conducted evenly throughout. A microwave oven temperature probe (not a glass thermometer) can be used to check that the temperature is high enough in the thickest part of the food.

Steaming

Vegetables are always best cooked in steam until tender. Boiling in water washes out many valuable nutrients.

The simplest utensil is a perforated trivet to hold the vegetables out of the boiling water in a pan, but there are many purpose-built steamers available.

Food Processors

Cooking your own food from the basic ingredients gives you the closest control over what you or your family eat. It allows you to keep the most closely to the food combining diet and it allows you to avoid all those additives which are needed to make processed foods palatable.

Fresh meat, vegetables and fruit do not need any elaborate processing. Neither do starchy meals based on rice, potatoes and vegetables. Wheat whole-meal bread from the supermarket is of high quality and can form the basis for up to half your starch meals.

The food combining diet does not include pastry or cakes and biscuits and so removes the need for a lot of elaborate processing equipment. A food mixer or processor is valuable if you plan to bake your own bread, and a grain mill is very useful for non-wheat flours for special diets.

Budget Meals

If you are providing meals on a low budget, remember the cost of wasted food as well as the cost of cooking. Buy food with as little waste as possible and trim it as little as necessary. Broad beans in their pods are mostly waste, but a solid cabbage is almost all good food. If you don't eat the fat, avoid the cheapest cuts of meat like belly pork, where you get little meat for your money, and examine the ends of a joint to select one without any thick fat layers. Always take the trouble to store food in the optimum conditions and use the most perishable food first. Don't buy more than you need, but shopping every day could take up a lot of time, so keep a balance.

Small amounts of ready-made meals and packaged foods can cost substantially more than fresh fruit and vegetables, and the cost of meat can far outweigh its value in the diet. If you have the time, then you don't need these ready-meals, and in many cases they take as long to prepare as fresh food.

There is no nutritional need to have a protein meal every day, and a lot of evidence that suggests that one protein meal every two or three days would be more healthy!

Low cost meals need not be monotonous with a wide range of dried herbs and spices available in the supermarkets. You use so little of these that you can afford to include them in the lowest budget meals.

If times are really hard then eat potatoes cooked in their skins, brown rice, sprouted beans and seeds, and a little olive oil together with herbs from your windowsill and spices. The cheapest vegetables, like carrots and cabbage are also the healthiest and require the minimum of cooking. Fresh wholemeal bread also remains excellent value for money.

Ready Meals

No 'modern' take-aways or cook/chill can match the ease of preparation, or the nutritional value of bread, salads and an olive oil dressing.

It is often cheaper to call in at the nearest supermarket for fresh fruit and vegetables for salad, than to buy them ready prepared.

A pressure cooker will often cook a protein meal, prepared from fresh ingredients, faster than it takes to thaw a frozen meal.

Food combining is the true modern lifestyle, based on a real knowledge of what is healthy and valuable in our lives.

Where you do need the ready prepared meals, it is often easier to select a starch based meal. But beware of excessive fat in sauces and fillings.

Vegetarian options often permit you to keep most closely to the food combining diet, but always remember that this is not a strait-jacket. It is the balance of the diet over weeks, months and years that determines your overall health.

On the occasion where you require a ready prepared meal simply select a low fat and low sugar meal.

Restaurants

There is nothing wrong in asking for what you want! We decide in advance whether a meal out is to be a protein meal or a starch meal - if you want to keep the price down, or make your choice easier, go for the starch meal!

You can ask for fresh fruit or vegetable dishes without any thickened sauces with either protein or starch meals.

If you select a protein meals, avoid battered fish, pies and pizzas. Plain fish is often the easiest as it is usually served with an unthickened sauce. Roasted and grilled meats can be requested without the potatoes or rice that usually accompany them and I always ask for extra vegetables instead. Fruit and cheese can round off a restaurant protein meal.

Starch meals can again start with fruit, or with garlic bread. If there are a selection of vegetables, I order these without a main course, together with potatoes or rice. I find the tastiest end to the meal is again, often fresh fruit.

Health Guide to Teenagers

As a teenager, you are going through a lot of changes. Your body is changing and growing. Have you noticed that every year, you can't seem to fit into your old shoes anymore? Or that your favorite jeans are now tighter or 3 inches too short? Your body is on its way to becoming its adult size.

Along with your physical changes, you are also becoming more independent. You are starting to make more choices about your life. You are relying less on your parents and more on yourself and your friends when making decisions. Some of the biggest choices that you face are those about your health.

Why should you care about your health? Well, there are lots of reasons—like feeling good, looking good, and getting stronger. Doing well in school, work, or other activities (like sports) is another reason. Believe it or not, these can all be affected by your health!

Healthy eating and being active now may also help prevent diabetes, high blood pressure, heart disease, osteoporosis, stroke, and some forms of cancer when you are older.

Some teenagers are not very physically active and some do not get the foods that their growing bodies need.

Now is the time to take charge of your health by eating better and being more physically active. Even small changes will help you look and feel your best!

Family Matters

Even if health problems run in your family, it doesn't mean that you will have the same problems . . .

To learn more about your health, start by looking at your family.

Are your parents, brothers, or sisters overweight? Do any of them have health problems related to their weight, such as type 2 diabetes? Your family's gene pool, eating habits, and activities can all play a role in your health and the way you look.

Type 2 diabetes is increasing in adolescents and teenagers who are overweight. Diabetes means that blood glucose (blood sugar) is too high. Diabetes is serious. It can hurt your eyes, kidneys, heart and blood vessels, gums, and teeth.

Even if members of your family have type 2 diabetes or other health problems, it doesn't mean that you will have the same problems. To lower your chances of developing them, eat healthy foods, get moving, and talk to your family or health care provider if you are concerned about your weight or health.

So, Where Do I Start?

The road to better health starts with good eating and physical activity habits. Being aware of your habits will help you learn where you need to make changes.

Do you normally watch a lot of TV or play a lot of video games? These activities can be relaxing, but you don't need to move much to do them. Spending too much time not moving around can make you feel tired and lazy, and lead to poor muscle tone. You can be active every day and still have time to do other things you enjoy, like playing video games!

Physical Activity—It Doesn't Have To Be A Chore! Being active means moving more every day. You can choose activities that are fun and do them on your own or with your friends.

Being more active will make you feel better and give you more energy. It can also help you think and concentrate better, which will help you in school or at work. Activity can help you feel less bored and depressed, and help you handle stress.

So don't wait—start today. Begin slowly and make small changes in your daily routine, like

spending less time in front of the TV

taking the stairs instead of the elevator

walking to school instead of taking the bus (or if you drive, parking further away on the school parking lot).

What you choose to do is up to you. Just pick something that you like to do and keep it up. Have fun while being active each day to stay healthy and fit. Remember, you don't have to give up the video games—just make sure that you also fit activity into your day.

Get Moving!

Walk—to school, to work, to your friend's house, to the mall.

Ride your bike.

Skateboard.

Rollerblade.

Walk with a friend or family member—make it "quality time"!

Play basketball.

Join a school sports team or club.

Walk the family dog. If you don't have one, find a neighbor who does.

Go dancing.

Go for a hike.

Go for a swim.

Wash the car.

Clean the house.

Mow the lawn.

(OK, the last three aren't fun, but your parents will appreciate you doing them!)

You Are What You Eat!

Take a look at your eating habits. What you eat, where you eat, and why you eat are important to your health. As a teen, you need to eat a variety of foods that give you the nutrients your growing body needs. Eating better and being more active can make you feel better and think more clearly.

What do you eat?

If you eat a lot of burgers and fries or pizza loaded with toppings—plus an extra helping of dessert—your diet is probably not balanced.

There's nothing wrong with eating these foods—you just need to eat smaller amounts and balance them with other foods.

Where do you usually eat?

If you eat in places such as your room or in front of the TV, you may want to change that habit. Eating while doing other things makes it easy to lose track of how much you've already eaten.

By eating meals and snacks at a table, you can pay more attention to what you're eating so that you don't overeat.

(If you want to snack while watching TV, take a small amount of food with you—such as a handful of pretzels or a couple of cookies—not the whole bag.)

Why do you eat?

To see if you need to change your eating habits, let's look at why you eat. For most people, reasons to eat are:

Time of day

Hunger

Food looks tempting

Everyone else is eating

Boredom, frustration, nervousness, or sadness

The best reason to eat is because your body tells you that you are hungry. If you are eating when you are not hungry, try doing something else to get food off of your mind. Call a friend, exercise, read, or work on a craft. These activities can help you to cut back on eating when you are feeling bored, upset, or stressed.

To improve your eating habits, try to eat the suggested number of servings from each food group in the Food Guide Pyramid.

The Food Guide Pyramid

Bread, cereal, rice, & pasta group (6-11 servings)

Vegetable group (3-5 servings)

Fruit group (2-4 servings)

Milk, yogurt, & cheese group (2-3 servings)

Meat, poultry, fish, dry beans, eggs, & nuts group (2-3 servings)

Fats, oils, & sweets (use sparingly)

Note: A range of servings is given for each group. The smaller number is for people who consume about 1,600 calories a day, such as inactive women. The larger number is for those who eat about 2,800 calories a day, such as teenage boys, active men, and very active women.

What Counts as a Serving?

Bread, Cereal, Rice, & Pasta Group

1 slice of bread
1 ounce of ready-to-eat cereal
½ cup of cooked cereal, rice, or pasta
Vegetable Group

1 cup of raw leafy vegetables
½ cup of other vegetables—cooked or chopped raw
¾ cup of vegetable juice
Fruit Group

1 medium apple, banana, or orange
½ cup of chopped, cooked, or canned fruit
¾ cup of fruit juice
Milk, Yogurt, & Cheese Group

1 cup of milk or yogurt
11/2 ounces of natural cheese
2 ounces of processed cheese (1 ounce is about the size of your thumb)

Meat, Poultry, Fish, Dry Beans, Eggs, & Nuts Group

2-3 ounces of cooked lean meat, poultry, or fish (3 ounces is about the size of a deck of cards)

½ cup of cooked dry beans or 1 egg counts as 1 ounce of lean meat. Two tablespoons of peanut butter or 1/3 cup of nuts counts as 1 ounce of meat.

For a Healthy Diet, Eat Daily— Breads, Cereals, Rice, and Pasta

(at least 6 servings daily)

Breads: whole-grain, whole-wheat, cracked wheat, multigrain, or oatmeal. (Go easy on high-fat spreads like butter.)

Cereals: whole-grain, hot and cold.

Rice and pasta: brown rice, whole-wheat or enriched pasta. (Try tomato sauces, which are lower in calories than cream sauces.)

Fruits
(at least 2 servings daily)
All kinds: fresh, canned, or frozen.

Vegetables
(at least 3 servings daily)
All kinds: fresh, canned, frozen, boiled, steamed, or baked.

Milk, Yogurt, and Cheese
(at least 2 servings daily)
Nonfat or lowfat milk, yogurt, and cheeses. (Foods from this group contain calcium, which is very important in a growing body.)

Meat, Poultry, Fish, Dry Beans, Eggs, and Nuts (at least 2 servings daily)

Meat, poultry, and fish: lean, skinless, broiled, roasted, or simmered instead of breaded and fried. (Or try dry beans and peas, which are lower in fat.)

Let's Talk About Health

Get moving. Activity can make you stronger and more flexible.

Eat healthy every day. Choose fruits, vegetables,

breads, cereals, lean meat, poultry, fish, dry beans, and lowfat or nonfat milk and cheeses.

Eat slowly. You will be able to tell when you are full before you eat too much.

Eat less fats, oils. and sweets. Butter, margarine, oils, candy, high-fat salad dressings, and soft drinks offer little or no protein, vitamins, or minerals.

Eat when you are hungry. Your body will tell you when it's hungry. Snacking is OK, but try to go for a variety of nutritious snacks. (See the ideas in the Snack Attack below.)

Snack Attack

Baked potato chips or tortilla chips with salsa Pretzels (lightly salted or unsalted)

Bagels with tomato sauce and lowfat cheese

Flavored rice cakes (like caramel or apple cinnamon)

Popcorn—air popped or lowfat microwave

Veggies with lowfat or fat-free dip

Lowfat cottage cheese topped with fruit or spread on whole-wheat crackers

Ice milk, lowfat frozen or regular yogurt (add skim milk, orange or pineapple juice, and sliced bananas or strawberries to make a lowfat milk shake)

Frozen fruit bars

Vanilla wafers, gingersnaps, graham crackers, animal crackers, fig bars, raisins

Angel food cake topped with strawberries or raspberries and lowfat whipped cream

String cheese

Staying Healthy and Happy

Being a teenager can be tough, and sometimes teens who are healthy try to lose weight even though they don't need to. You may feel a lot of pressure to look a certain way. Acting on this pressure may lead to eating disorders like anorexia nervosa or bulimia nervosa.

Anorexia nervosa is a form of self-starvation where a person does not eat enough food to keep healthy and does not maintain a healthy weight.

Bulimia nervosa is when a person eats a lot of food and then vomits or uses other methods, such as fasting or overexercising, to avoid gaining weight after overeating.

If you would like to learn more about eating disorders, see the list of resources at the end of this booklet.

If you are concerned about your eating habits or the way you look, it's important to talk to someone you trust. Try talking to a parent, friend, doctor, teacher, or counselor at your school.

Being happy with who you are and what you look like is important for a healthy body and mind. You don't have to be an athlete, supermodel, or movie star to like who you are and to stay fit and healthy.

You can take charge of your health by making small changes in your eating and physical activity habits. These changes will help you feel and look better now and be healthier for the rest of your life!

CHAPTER 5

FOOD ALLERGIES & EATING DISORDERS

Egg, Milk & Wheat Allergies

There is no treatment for food allergy other than avoiding the food in question, but this isn't always as simple as it sounds. If you are allergic to eggs, for instance, you have to avoid everything containing eggs. Besides carefully checking the labels of all commercially prepared foods, this also means speaking to your doctor about vaccines made with egg residues, which include injections for flu and yellow fever.

If you are highly allergic and have had an anaphylactic reaction in the past, avoiding the food in question can be a matter of life or death. Constant vigilance is required because the smallest amount of the allergen can set off a reaction. Just 1/44,000 of a peanut kernel can trigger a reaction in someone highly allergic to peanuts. Less sensitive people may be able to tolerate small amounts of the allergic food. Still, it's wise to avoid these foods altogether and remove them from your home. Here's what to look for:

Egg Allergies

Check labels of food products for the following offending ingredients: "egg," "egg white," "dried egg" or "albumin." And avoid these products:

- Cakes and cookies, unless homemade with egg-free recipes using commercially available egg replacements. Make sure you buy "replacements" not "substitutes," which can contain egg white.
- Chocolates, marshmallows and fondants
- Soups containing egg noodles (including alphabet soup), or any other soup made with eggs
- Mayonnaise
- Custards, puddings, ice cream, filling for cream pies including coconut, lemon and pumpkin pies
- Eggnog and egg creams
- French toast, fritters and pancakes

- Muffins, rolls, bagels, donuts, or any bread that contains egg. (Most breads do not contain eggs, but check ingredient lists carefully to be sure.)
- Meatloaf and other meat, chicken or fish dishes made with egg or dipped in batter containing eggs
- Meringues
- Pretzels
- Egg substitutes
- Sauces and salad dressing containing eggs: hollandaise, dressing for Caesar salad, Russian dressing, mayonnaise-based dressings

Milk Allergies

Check labels carefully for the following ingredients: "milk," "whey," "dried milk solids," "casein," "lactalbumin," "sodium caseinate," "potassium caseinate," "calcium caseinate," "butter," "cheese," "margarine" and "curds." Do not eat any of the following foods:

- Milk
- Cream
- Yogurt
- Lactaid
- Acidophilus milk
- Ice cream and ice milk, sherbets made with milk or frozen yogurt
- Cream sauces and soups, white sauces
- Butter or margarine (except parve)
- Cheese
- Baked goods made with milk, including breads
- Mashed potatoes and other vegetables prepared with milk, cheese, butter or cream
- Instant cocoa, breakfast mixes and cereals containing dried milk.

Wheat Allergies

Check labels to be sure that even small amounts of wheat are not present in the list of ingredients. Words that indicate there's wheat include "wheat," "flour," "wheat germ," "wheat starch," "bran," "modified food starch," "graham flour," "farina" and "semolina." Avoid these products:

- Bread, crackers and other baked goods (except those made without wheat; rye bread and cornbread usually contain wheat)
- Most cereals
- All pasta and noodles made from wheat
- Fried chicken and other fried foods dipped in bread crumbs or flour made from wheat
- Meatloaf and other foods containing bread crumbs, cracker crumbs, cereal or other forms of wheat. This includes most sausages, hot dogs and some cold cuts.
- Sauces and gravies thickened with flour
- Prepared salad dressings thickened with flour or other forms of wheat
- Pancakes, waffles and fritters What People Mistake For Food Allergies

There's a lot of confusion about food allergies. Often a symptom related to the ingestion of particular food has nothing to do with the immune system and, therefore, is not an allergic reaction. Indigestion? Maybe. Lactose intolerance? Possibly. Food sensitivity? Could be. Several conditions can be mistaken for an allergic reaction.

- Lactose intolerance — Some people cannot tolerate dairy products because they lack the enzyme, lactase, needed to digest lactose (milk sugar). If lactose intolerance is your problem, you probably develop gas, cramps or diarrhea when you consume dairy foods. Some people are affected only when they have larger than usual amounts of these foods, and most lactose-intolerant people can tolerate hard cheeses, yogurt and sour cream without developing symptoms. Lactose intolerance can be diagnosed with a blood test.
- Asthma — People with asthma can develop attacks after eating foods containing sulfites, additives used to keep food looking fresh and to retard mold growth. Although the U.S. Food and Drug Administration now bans the use of sulfite sprays on fresh fruits and vegetables, they still are used in dried fruit and other foods. Sulfites also develop naturally in wine during fermentation.
- Celiac disease — In this uncommon condition, cells lining the small intestine are damaged by gluten, a protein in wheat and other grains. The main symptoms are gas and bloating. Celiac disease usually develops in

childhood but can begin at any age. If you or your child is affected, you will have to avoid breads and other foods that contain gluten. That can be a challenge, since many foods contain hidden grains.

- Reactions to specific foods — Some people can't eat beans, peas, broccoli or cabbage without developing uncomfortable intestinal gas. Others develop indigestion and diarrhea after eating mushrooms or drinking certain wines. While the symptoms sometimes are confused with food allergies, they aren't caused by an allergic reaction.
- Reactions to food additives — In susceptible people, the food additive monosodium glutamate (MSG), which often is used in Chinese food, can bring on symptoms that include dizziness, sweating, ringing in the ears and a feeling of faintness. This "Chinese restaurant syndrome" actually is an intolerance to MSG, and not a food allergy. In rare instances, another food additive, yellow dye number 5, can cause hives.
- Food poisoning — Nausea, vomiting and diarrhea caused by food poisoning or by an infection, such as gastrointestinal flu, can be mistaken for a food allergy. Food poisoning stems from contamination with bacteria or other microorganisms, while gastrointestinal flu is a viral infection that affects the digestive system. A bout of food poisoning mistakenly labeled as an allergy can affect dietary choices for years to come.
- Histamine toxicity — You can develop an allergylike reaction to foods containing histamine, a natural substance involved in the allergic process. Foods high in histamine include cheese and some wines. Certain kinds of fish, particularly tuna and mackerel, are high in histamine, but the high levels may be due to contamination if the fish wasn't properly refrigerated.

Eating Disorders

What is disordered eating, and how can it be prevented? Normal, healthy eating behavior may be defined as when a person eats when she or he is hungry, and stops eating when full. That is, the person is aware of and responds appropriately to hunger and satiety cues. Of course, all of us can recall a time when we have eaten past our natural fullness point, or have skipped a meal even when hungry. This does not mean everyone has disordered ,eating, although variations of this problem are extremely common. It is only when an individual consistently ignores feelings of hunger or fullness and this pattern of behavior becomes usual for them that the person may be said to have disordered eating. "Disordered eating" covers a broad spectrum of eating behavior including eating disorders, while the term "eating disorder" is defined quite specifically by diagnostic criteria.

Some possible causes of disordered eating include negative body image, low self-esteem, peer pressure, and lack of information about how eating and dieting can affect health. In order to prevent these problems, we must look at what is believed to cause them. Both of the topics mentioned above note that eating disorders fill a need for the individual. For example, eating is a self-soothing activity. It is quite possible that a "cause" of overeating might be that the child has not learned any other way to soothe himself or calm down when he is upset. Similarly, a teen girl might find her need for attention met when she loses weight after being on a diet. Like all dysfunctions, the principle of "overdetermination" applies. There are many causes and predisposing factors, which in combination can influence a person to adopt a disordered eating pattern. Some would say that just being a member (especially female) of western society, is a predisposing factor. Foreyt and Goodrick in their book "Living Without Dieting" point out that western culture is a "lookist" culture, overemphasizing appearance and underemphasizing human qualities. Lookism, like racism or sexism, defines people by external characteristics that have nothing to do with a person's real abilities. Most young people are strongly influenced by media images which associate unrealistic thinness with beauty, sexiness, money, power and happiness. Lookism is not talked about, but is a very real social force.

Recent research shows that body dissatisfaction is the single strongest predictor of eating disorder symptomolgy (Phelps, Johnston and Augustyniak, 1999)*. Helping teen girls (and boys) recognize the positive attributes of their physical appearance may be the most effective prevention strategy we have. This approach increases feelings of self-efficacy, helping them feel "OK". It also helps reduce the internalization of the unnatural "ideal" body standard, and lets them realize that each person expresses their own inner beauty differently. It is important to understand that young people are bombarded with hundreds of messages about attractiveness every day. All influential adults play a role in letting kids know what is "right" with their looks. Adults who are not comfortable with their own appearance may be most hard pressed to send positive messages to teens.

Girls and women are more at risk than boys and men, probably due to unreasonable expectations for female body shape and distorted expressions of female beauty portrayed in the media. Debra Waterhouse's excellent book "Like Mother Like Daughter" traces the legacy of dieting and disordered eating through the generations, while offering strategies to break this destructive cycle.

Boys and men are not exempt from the pressures to modify their bodies. Unfortunately, exploitation of men based on appearance is on the increase, and this is likely to result in greater numbers of males with disordered eating. Magazines covers of men with abdominal muscle definition few can ever achieve are found in every check out stand, next to the women's magazines featuring impossibly thin but full busted female models. Young people view these pictures as the standard of attractiveness and try hard to measure up.

Sports can have a mixed effect on body image as well. Studies show that girls who participate in sports have higher scores for self esteem and are less likely to be victimized by others. However, it is well known that certain sports which emphasize thinness, like gymnastics, dance and figure skating, put girls at higher risk. For boys, wrestling can contribute to dysfunctional eating behaviors and purging in order to attain/maintain an unnatural weight. Parents and coaches need to give healthy, non-diet messages to teen athletes. Coaches especially have a strong influence on whether an athlete learns to be their best with the body shape and size they have, or ends up wasting precious mental and physical energy on artificial weight goals. Dieting has a negative impact on sports performance. Good sports nutrition, on the other hand, can enhance performance on and off the playing field.

Prevention Strategies

Parents, teachers and coaches: Your example matters! Practice healthy eating behaviors. Eat when you get up in the morning, and eat every 4 hours or so throughout the day. This will help your body get on schedule, so that you will experience hunger on a regular basis. Stop eating when you are full! Your body knows better than you do how to maintain a healthy weight.

Coaches: Your actions and your words are more important than you know! Many cases of eating disorders in athletes start when coaches tell them that weight loss will improve performance. Read up on sports nutrition. Consider getting a registered dietitian to speak to team members and parents.

Mothers: Be aware of your own weight issues. Dieting is not "normal", despite what media influences may say. If your teen is experiencing difficulties, don't blame yourself. Instead, be part of the solution by treating your own body with respect.

All influential adults: Listen to what you say! Our language has incorporated many myths that you may spread unconsciously. Were you "good" today by eating salad, but "bad" yesterday when you ate a brownie? There are no good and bad foods. All foods can fit into a healthy diet. Talk to kids about what really is good and bad, and share your values with them.

Help children learn how to get their needs met. Teach them how to ask for what they need. Many experts believe that disordered eating behaviors are a language used by people who don't have the words to say "that makes me mad" or "I feel hurt."

Make a point of recognizing kids' attractive physical features. Many times we spoil a compliment by adding "if you didn't have such heavy legs" or some such negative remark. Praise really won't spoil kids, even when it comes to appearance! Criticism will not help them lose weight, it will only damage their self esteem.

Teach critical thinking skills. Help kids think problems through. Does it really make sense to think that going on a diet will solve the problem?

Avoid "horror" stories of anorexia or bulimia. Scaring kids usually doesn't work and may teach dysfunctional behavior.

Help children relax. If relaxation means sitting in front of the TV eating chips, the child is being set up for a weight problem as well as missing out on skills needed to reduce stress. Use physical activity as a stress release. You know it's working if you can say you had fun!

Exercise in moderation. Physical activity is for fun and health, not to burn calories or achieve a certain percent body fat.

Examine cultural values. Do you really think its necessary to look a certain way in order to be happy? Promote size acceptance as part of the natural diversity of human beings.

Accept your own body. It is just as hard for adults to resist negative media messages as it is for kids, especially since we've been hearing them longer! Helping kids can be a reason to help ourselves.

Develop "learned hardiness". Kids can learn to roll with the punches and resist influences that depress or discourage them. Encourage activities that build character.

Avoid dieting! Research shows that most eating disorders started with a diet. Diets don't work! See the resource list below for weight management strategies that do work

Nutrition for Athletes

Nutrition: "those properties of food that build sound bodies and promote health; a balanced diet containing adequate amounts of the essential nutritional elements that the body must have to function normally."

Nutrition by any other name still means the same thing...nourishment, sustenance, FOOD! As an athlete, you know that nutrition plays a key role in your performance. But often, this component of training is misunderstood. There is a wealth of nutritional information out there and it can get pretty confusing.

What is the best training diet? High or low carbohydrate? High or low protein? Low fat or no fat? One popular diet advises a dietary regimen of , 40% carbohydrate, 30% protein, and 30% fat at each of three small meals (about

500 calories each) and two snacks (about 100 calories each) per day. Is this the best diet for optimum athletic performance? Without delving into a lot of scientific lingo, let me shed some light on these ideas.

The favored fuel for exercise is carbohydrate. It is stored in the form of glycogen in your muscles and liver glycogen. You cannot train or compete well on a low carbohydrate, low calorie diet. You need to eat enough calories and carbohydrate to maintain muscle and liver glycogen stores. The above diet is only about 1700 calories per day; much too low for the average athlete training several hours a week. Your body stores only about 1600-2100 calories of carbohydrate in your muscles, liver, and blood. This is the energy equivalent of a 150 pound athlete running 15-18 miles. When your muscle glycogen is depleted, you "hit the wall" and feel overwhelmingly fatigued and ready to quit. When your liver glycogen is depleted you "bonk" (feel uncoordinated, light-headed, weak, unable to concentrate) because inadequate glucose is available to the brain. The bottom line is that the majority of your diet should come from carbohydrate sources to insure adequate fuel for training.

Let's move on to protein. Contrary to popular belief, exercise, not extra dietary protein, builds muscle. Today's popular high protein diets will not provide enough carbohydrate to fuel your muscles to allow you to exercise hard enough to meet your potential. Depending on your athletic goals your protein needs range from 0.55 to 0.81 grams of protein per pound of body weight per day, or about 80 - 122 grams per day for a 150 pound athlete. Serious weight lifters are at the upper end of the range. A diet too high in protein may make you too full to eat adequate amounts of carbohydrate to fuel your muscles. High protein diets may also promote dehydration through excess urination when waste products from protein metabolism are excreted. Finally, a high protein intake may promote a high fat intake, because many high protein foods are also high in fat.

And what about fat in your diet? How much fat do you need? Most athletes tend to err on the conservative side when it comes to fat. We avoid it like we avoid missing a workout. Fat has become the bad guy. Just about any food these days is available in a "fat free" version. Truth is, our bodies need some fat. A diet too low in fat can impair exercise performance. Fat is an essential part of hormones, cell membranes, and the nervous system. Fat is needed for the absorption of fat soluble vitamins A, D, E, and K. Perhaps the most obvious function of fat in your diet is that it makes you feel full and satisfied after eating. Without some fat in your diet, you may feel hungry all the time.

So what does all this mean? The best training diet is composed of 60-70% carbohydrate, 10-20% protein, and 20-25% fat. Although supplements may be convenient, there is no need to consume fancy protein powders or supplements. Save your money and spend it on good, healthful food. Eat plenty of whole grain breads, cereal, rice, pasta, potatoes, and fresh fruits/vegetables for carbohydrates; dried beans/peas, lean meats, and low fat dairy products for protein; and moderate amounts of fat from primarily unsaturated sources (olive/canola/peanut oils, nuts/seeds, avocados, light margarine/salad dressing). And remember to drink plenty of non-caffeinated fluids.

Now let's put this in more practical terms. The average calorie needs for a competitive endurance athlete training about seven hours a week is at least 3500 calories for a male and 2800 calories for a female. This is a general guideline, so don't worry about counting calories. Be more concerned with getting a balanced intake of a variety of healthful foods. The following is a sample 3000 calorie training diet to give you an idea of the appropriate amount of food to eat to keep you well-fueled for optimum performance:

Breakfast: 2 cups whole grain cereal 1 cup skim milk 1 slice whole wheat toast 1 Tbsp. Light Margarine 1 Tbsp. Jam 1 cup orange juice 1 banana

Morning Snack: 1 cup plain low-fat yogurt 1 cup strawberries sprinkled with 1 tsp sugar 2 graham cracker sheets

Lunch: Turkey Sandwich 2 slices whole wheat bread 3 ounces turkey 1 Tbsp. Light Mayonnaise Lettuce and tomato 1 ounce baked chips or pretzels 1 cup grapes 1 cup raw baby carrots

Afternoon Snack: 1 cup skim milk 3 fig cookie bars

Dinner: 1.5 cups cooked pasta 1 cup tomato sauce mixed with ½ cup cottage cheese 4 Tbsp Parmesan Cheese 3 cups mixed vegetable salad 2 Tbsp Light Salad Dressing 1 slice Garlic Bread

Evening Snack: 1 cup Light Frozen Yogurt

Total Calories: 3000
Total CHO: 475 g (~63% kcals)
Total fat: 72 g (~22% kcals)
Total pro: 116g (~15% kcals)

Food is fuel. But food is also pleasure. Your body is pretty smart. If you eat a variety of wholesome foods most of the time, then you can afford to fit in your favorite dessert or gooey treat occasionally. All foods can fit into your diet. There is no such thing as a "good" or "bad" food, only better food choices. If you fuel your body properly, then it will be better equipped to help you meet your athletic potential.

The Basics of Muscle Recovery Post Workout

By Syd Johnston RD/LD/CSCS

There are many factors to consider when you're trying to decide what to do for post-exercise muscle recovery. Here is a thumbnail sketch of how to plan for your recovery, which begins before you work out.

Before Exercise

The best way to make your muscle recovery plan effective is to go into your work out in a well-nourished state to prevent depletion of energy, water, and nutrient stores. Our first consideration, water, is the fluid medium in which virtually every biochemical reaction in the body must occur. The body is approximately 65-70% water, and skeletal muscle is on the high end at 70% water. When we become dehydrated our performance and physical health become compromised. Adequate fluid balance (hydration) is essential for optimal performance and for effective recovery from training or exercise.

Eat a carbohydrate rich meal with adequate protein and fat; one that is agreeable to you and if prior to competition, will not react adversely with pre-competition jitters. Timing is important as well, so you probably will not want to eat any closer than two hours to ninety minutes prior to exercise while maintaining hydration through liberal consumption of water and/or sports drink before competition.

During Exercise

It is essential that during exercise, especially in the heat, 4-8 oz. of water or sports drink beverage be consumed regularly (every 15-30 minutes) to prevent dehydration. Even with regular intervals of rehydration fluid losses will still occur.(1) Post-training you may need to consume anywhere between a pint to as much as a gallon or more of water or sports drink depending on the intensity of training and the environmental conditions in which you may have exercised.

Any athlete who has ever exercised in the heat for a period of more than 30 minutes knows what the repercussions are for lack of proper hydration: muscle cramping, nausea, dizziness, heat stroke, and possibly even a heart attack if the exerciser or athlete is not acclimated and is seriously dehydrated. Any one of these is enough to throw a wrench in anybody's post-work out muscle recovery plan and might even make you wish you had not gone out at all. So my advice is, drink up!

After Exercise

For most people, the first order of business comes about very naturally: we rush to find the nearest source of water whether it be a fluid-filled backpack, water fountain or bottle of water or sports drink. After quenching your thirst your next thoughts might turn to replenishing your body with carbs, protein, and electrolytes. Another consideration might be how to best recover from delayed onset muscle soreness (DOMS).

Basic guidelines for rehydration after exercise are that for every pound of weight you lose from a work out, 2-3 cups of fluid should be consumed to replace it. Weigh yourself prior to exercise and again after exercise to determine how much weight you have lost. It is virtually all fluid weight lost through sweat, water droplets in expired air, and insensible losses. The amount of weight lost is the amount of fluid you need to consume. Water or sports drinks are the best fluid-replacement choices.

In prolonged exercise in the heat sweat loss may deplete up to 13 to 17 grams of sodium in a day, which is about 8-10 grams more sodium than is consumed in a typical American diet. Potassium loss through exercise usually is negligible except under the most extreme conditions such as endurance training in desert heat. Consumption of fruit such as oranges, honey dew melon, or raisins will provide sufficient repletion of any potassium lost in a typical one to two hour workout. If exercise is prolonged extra sodium may need to be consumed. This can be done by consuming an oral rehydration solution (sports drink) or simply by adding some salt to your food; about one teaspoon will do.

The consumption of carbohydrates post-work out is vitally important for restoration of lost glycogen. Glycogen is the storage form of glucose which is derived from the carbohydrate-containing foods we eat. It is the major energy source from which muscle derives its power during exercise. An athlete who trains aerobically at high intensity for an hour or more can decrease liver glycogen by 55% and can significantly decrease glycogen levels in the exercised muscles such as the quads and hamstrings in the case of a runner. Activities of high intensity for a minute or more with short periods of rest can dramatically decrease muscle glycogen content in the exercised muscles. Examples of such activities are ice hockey, soccer, track running drills, or moderate to high volume resistance training with short rest periods.

Carbohydrate needs post-work out vary from person to person and are dependent upon intensity, duration of exercise, and of course, body size. In general, for every hour of exercise 50-75 grams of carbohydrate should be consumed up to a total of 500 grams post workout. Foods such as white rice, pasta, grapes, raisins, bananas, or any food that is high in carbohydrates and low in fat and fiber are excellent choices. Foods high in fiber like apples, pears, tomatoes ,bell peppers, squash, beans, whole grains, and/or high in fat like candy bars, ice cream, peanut butter, whole milk should not be eaten post-work out because they will delay gastric emptying and thereby prevent rapid repletion of muscle glycogen.

Protein may also be used as an energy source, especially if the athlete is following a low carbohydrate diet or is near the end of an intense competition or training session and his/her glycogen stores are near depletion. When glycogen stores become depleted or are near depletion the body will begin using free amino acids as a source of energy. This inhibits anabolism, which is contrary to the goals of athletes. In terms of exercise, the longer you exercise, as in the case of an endurance runner, it is very likely that amino acids will be catabolized (broken down) to glucose to supply energy to working muscles as well as to sustain necessary metabolic processes. This can occur when a person either has not adequately fueled-up on carbohydrate and fat, or has exercised past the point provided by stored glycogen and it becomes easier for the body to utilize the free amino acids than to liberate and oxidize stored glycogen and lipids.

Practically speaking, break up your protein intake into four meals per day, with one of those meals being your post-workout meal. For example, based on the protein needs of an endurance athlete weighing 82 kg discussed below, each meal should contain roughly 25-30 grams protein, including the post-workout meal. The strength training individual weighing 82 kg will need between 30-41 grams protein post workout with the same provision of 4 meals day with roughly similar amounts protein per meal.

Time your post-workout meal based on adage: "the sooner the better". Typically consumption of carbohydrates and protein should occur within 30 to 90 minutes post-exercise to achieve the greatest recovery benefits.

Your Diet Every Day

In order to keep up with the demand of the body on amino acids it is recommended that endurance athletes, due to their long bouts of exercise, consume 1.2-1.4 grams of protein per kilogram body weight per day (g/kg/d). For example, a 180 pound (lb.) person weighs about 82 kg (1 kg = 2.2 lbs.). This means a 180 lb. person would need from 98-114 g. of protein per day to keep up with protein synthesis, energy demands, and other physiologic stresses. Of course, these recommendations and others to follow are contingent on the intake of adequate calories and portions of carbohydrate and fat in the diet to provide for your body's primary energy needs.

The needs of strength athletes are slightly different from their endurance counterparts. The demands of strength training do not typically involve amino acid oxidation from the skeletal muscle, rather it is the trauma placed upon the myofibrils of the skeletal muscle which are the cause of increased protein needs. During strength training, if the intensity level is high enough, micro-tears will occur in the actin-myosin filaments, which are the basic unit of muscle contraction. These tears are also responsible for a phenomenon known as Delayed Onset Muscle Soreness (DOMS), which is the pain we feel a day or two after a hard training session.

In order for our body to synthesize proteins to repair the damaged tissue from an intense workout it is suggested that you consume from a range of 1.4-2.0g/kg/day of protein. So using the example of the 180 lb. person, about 115-164 g protein per day should be consumed by this particular strength athlete.

One ounce of lean meat, fish, or two egg whites contains 7 grams of complete protein (all essential amino acids available in necessary proportions for growth) . One cup (8 ounces) of milk contains 8 grams of complete protein . Vegetables in general contain 2 grams of incomplete protein. Breads, grains, and cereals provide 3 grams incomplete protein per serving. And as you may have guessed complete protein sources are better protein choices to support tissue-building and repair.

If you're a vegetarian the variety of protein sources available to you can be just as beneficial as those available to non-vegetarians depending on the strictness of your vegetarian diet. Lacto-ovo- and fish-eating vegetarians have more options of foods that are already complete proteins in milk products, fish, and the most efficient of all proteins, eggs and egg whites, all of which can be wonderful post-work out foods. Vegans can get adequate protein from consuming beans, soy milk, whole grains and vegetables. Of course, post-work out you will want to consume the majority of your carbs prior to eating any fibrous vegetables due to their ability to slow down glucose entry into the bloodstream.

Strategy For Recovery

Evidence that treatment with modalities such as ice pack or heat pad, electrical stimulation, massage, and further eccentric training post-exercise will enhance muscle recovery from DOMS are equivocal at best. So far, a dearth of studies exist showing that any one of these therapies is any more effective than the other in speeding up recovery time from DOMS. Your best bet to recover from DOMS is to cool down post-exercise by doing a few light reps on the muscle group worked or to jog or ride at a relaxed pace and then stretch for 5 or more minutes to help your muscles clear out lactic acid and other by-products that build up over the course of a work out. And of course you will want to consume a carbohydrate-rich meal from grains or breads and fruit with adequate protein and fluid to start the recovery proce

Eating Disorder

Anorexia and bulimia have destroyed thousands of lives and placed the victims in a mental prison that is endured 24 hours a day, every day. The clinical definitions of these disorders are as follows:

Anorexia Nervosa

A. Refusal to maintain body weight at or above a minimally normal weight for age and height.
B. Intense fear of gaining weight or becoming fat, even though underweight.
C. Disturbance in the way in which one's body weight or shape is experienced, undue influence of body weight or shape of self-evaluation, or denial of the seriousness of the current low body weight.
D. Amenorrhea in postmenarchal women, that is, the absence of at least three consecutive menstrual cycles.

Bulimia Nervosa

A. Recurrent episodes of binge eating. An episode of binge eating is characterized by both of the following:

1. Eating, in a discrete period of time, an amount of food that is definitely larger than most people would eat during a similar period of time and under similar circumstances, and
2. A sense of lack of control over eating during the episode (e.g., a feeling that one cannot stop eating or control what or how much one is eating).

B. Recurrent inappropriate compensatory behavior in order to prevent weight gain, such as self-induced vomiting; misuse of laxatives, diuretics, enemas, or other medications; fasting; or excessive exercise.

C. The binge eating and inappropriate compensatory behaviors both occur, on average, at least twice a week for three months.

D. Self-evaluation is unduly influenced by body shape and weight.

E. The disturbance does not occur exclusively during episodes of anorexia nervosa.

(Taken from the Diagnostic and Statistical Manual, Fourth Edition.)

While these definitions give objective definitions that the medical, psychological, and insurance communities can agree on, eating disorders exist on a continuum of disordered eating practices. Someone could be suffering in the beginning stages of one of these disorders and not clearly fall into these definitions. The earlier eating disorders are discovered and treated, the better the outcome and the fewer the heartbreaks. Below are listed other signs and symptoms of these disorders that could be early warning signals of a developing problem:

Anorexia

- Undue attention to counting fat grams or calories.
- Refusal to eat a certain category of food (ex.meat, fat, sugar) that arises for no known reason.
- Obsessive attention to weight.
- Lack of desire to participate in social functions involving food (isolation).
- Relentless pursuit of activity and exercise.
- Deceptive actions around eating (ex. hiding food, lying about food eaten).

- Food rituals, such as cutting food into tiny portions, re-heating food multiple times, insistence upon eating at an exact time or refusal to eat after a certain time.
- Constant comments about being fat, feeling fat .. despite excessive thinness.
- Increase in depressive personality traits.
- Development of obsessive behaviors in other areas; such as cleanliness, study habits, organization, etc.
- Comments placing foods into "good' and "bad" categories and then pursuing "perfection" in food selection.
- Perfectionist goals and attitudes in other areas of life.
- Wearing of loose clothes to hide weight loss.
- Increased interest in information about food, nutrition, weight, etc. Consuming the same foods day after day in order to maintain a "safe" and "controlled" intake.
- Skipping of meals, sometimes eating very little, or fasting for days.
- Pale skin or other changes in the condition of skin. Loss of hair on the scalp, while growth of downy like hair increases on arms, back or stomach.
- Complaints of being excessively cold.
- Signs of increased muscle weakness and general lethargy.

Bulimia

Since bulimia often begins with restrictive practices, many of the early warning signs and symptoms will be similar to those for anorexia. In addition the following indicators may be apparent:

- Frequent trips to the bathroom following meals.
- Evidence of purging in and around the bathroom.
- Indications that laxatives, diuretics , or enemas are being used.
- Signs of secretive eating or bingeing.
- Dramatic fluctuations between restriction and overeating accompanied by weight fluctuations of 10 pounds or more.
- Evidence of self-induced vomiting, i.e. blood shot eyes, "chipmunk cheeks", or knuckle scarring.

- Presence of other impulse control behaviors such as stealing, shoplifting, or substance abuse.

The development of any one of these behaviors, attitudes, or symptoms does not indicate that one is in a full blown eating disorder. However, it may be an indication that the person is at risk. The greater the number of these early indicators that are apparent, the greater the risk.

What are the causes of these eating disorders?

There are no simple answers to this question. The causes are diverse, complex, and numerous. We may never know all of the contributing factors. We do know some of the ingredients that seem to be part of the recipe that makes one vulnerable to becoming in bondage to an eating disorder. When only a few of the "ingredients" are present, the person may only exist in some level of disordered eating and never move into a clinically diagnosable eating disorder.

One fundamental circumstance that is prevalent among those suffering from eating disorders is that they come from societies where thinness is prized and promoted as the ideal. In the United States it is estimated that 70% of all girls and young women have "felt fat" to the point of going on a diet before the age of 21. Thinness is equated with achieving happiness, success and all good things in much of our media and advertisements. It has been my experience that very few people swing into eating disorders without having participated in some form of dieting or restriction. This often opens the door to undertaking other artificial, disordered measures to achieve a weight that is unnatural and a body that is unobtainable through rational means.

Participation in a sport that emphasizes a leanness-performance connection or that involves wearing scant clothing seems to create an environment that can predispose one to the development of an eating disorder. Research indicates that anywhere between 30 - 70% of girls and young women that participate in sports such as dance, gymnastics, or track engage in some form of disordered eating practice. There has been an increasing awareness of the occurrence of eating disorders among males involved in certain sports such as wrestling and long distance running. Research into eating disorders among males is lacking.

Eating disorders often develop as a means of getting needs met. There are two age categories when a young woman appears to be vulnerable from this standpoint. These age groups are 13-14yr. olds and 17-18 yr. olds. These are ages when one deals extensively with self-esteem and body-esteem issues, identity and self-determination issues, and major changes (such as going into junior high or leaving home for college or work). Disordered eating behaviors may evolve as a mechanism to deal with stress, achieve "control" at a time in life when other circumstances seem uncertain and unmanageable, or it can be a form of rebellion (anorexia is often referred to as a "hunger strike"). These behaviors can serve the "purpose" of providing a way of gaining attention and a unique identity for oneself. As one recovers, healthier coping methods are learned to get needs met and to deal with difficult feelings, thoughts, and circumstances.

There is research ongoing to discover if there might be a genetic component to the development of eating disorders. While the jury is still out on the final verdict, there does seem to be evidence that many of those with eating disorders come from families where there has been substance abuse. This also could be evidence of the impact that family dysfunction could have in this area.

The Medical and Psychological Consequences of Eating Disorders

The medical consequences of these eating disorders can vary from the most common (menstrual irregularities or amenorrhea) to death. It has been estimated that the long-term death rate for those afflicted with anorexia or bulimia can be as high as 20 - 30%. Electrolyte deficiencies can arise that may cause nausea, fainting, muscle cramps, and damage to the heart muscle. In the worse case scenario, the cardiac muscle will cease functioning and death will occur. Other organs, such as the liver or kidney, may be damaged. With bulimics or purging anorexics, the esophagus may become irritated or ruptured. Laxative abuse can lead to irritable bowel disease or create an addiction to laxatives. Vitamin and mineral deficiencies can emerge from starvation or purging that can bring about problems with eyesight, skin, hair loss, osteoporosis, or easily fractured bones. The longer this disorder prevails, the more likely that some undesirable medical consequence will occur.

From a psychological perspective it can sometimes be difficult to decipher what problems have arisen as a result of the eating disorder verses what psychological conditions might have been a precursor to the development of anorexia or bulimia. This is particularly true with the most prevalent psychological state, depression. With severe nutritional imbalances and starvation, depression is a general consequence. Therefore, these issues may need to be addressed prior to determining if there was an undiagnosed depression that contributed to the eating disorder. Brain functioning may be affected, which is exhibited by the lack of ability to concentrate. Obsessive and compulsive behavior traits may be exhibited for the first time, or there may be a worsening of obsessive/compulsive disorders. In general, most of the psychological consequences will not be permanent in nature. Therapy and appropriate medications are very affective in addressing these issues.

Treatment Options

The first step in determining where to begin to with treatment options is with a medical exam by a physician that understands eating disorders. This is essential to determine if the individual is medically stable. If not, a medical hospitalization would be advisable before pursuing other options.

An unfortunate but undeniable fact is that most people must make treatment decisions with finances in mind. Most insurance companies are tightening the reigns on what they approve for residential or inpatient treatment of eating disorders. For this reason, it is recommend that outpatient treatment be examined as the next course to be pursued. This generally consists of the client working with a team of professionals that is made up of a physician, a nutrition therapist (registered dietitian), a psychologist or other mental health specialist, and, often, a psychiatrist. It is important that the team members are all experienced in the treatment of eating disorders and that they are willing and able to maintain effective communication with each other. Sometimes group therapy is also offered in this setting.

Inpatient treatment is often offered within the context of a psychiatric unit at a medical center or at a separate facility. These programs often treat other psychiatric and mental conditions. They may or may not specialize in eating disorders which may be advisable if there are other diagnoses present (i.e. substance abuse or sexual abuse issues).

Residential treatment centers offer intensive treatment in a non-hospital setting that allows for more freedom than inpatient. This type of treatment may last from as little as two weeks up to several months in duration. These facilities usually specialize in the treatment of eating disorders. Most often, the family of the patient becomes involved at some point during the treatment process. There is a complete team on staff and a variety of therapies are offered. This may include art therapy, body image work, and group therapy in addition to intensive individual therapy.

How can loved cnes support someone suffering from an eating disorder?

If you suspect someone you care about is dealing with an eating disorder and has not acknowledged their problem, it is best to approach them with evidence and not conjecture. Someone who is in denial abut their eating disorder is also more likely to listen to concerns if more than one person approaches them with those concerns at the same time. This is sometimes referred to as an "intervention". This should occur in a calm, loving, non-judgmental setting.

You can enhance your ability to support your loved one by learning as much as possible about eating disorders. This may prevent you from unknowingly offering simplistic advice for a complicated mental disorder. Many a sufferer has been alienated from those trying to help them by hearing statements like "just eat" or "that behavior is so disgusting." Suggested resources are listed below.

Helping ferret out treatment options, lending a listening ear or planning diversions to help make life less focused on the eating disorder can be caring ways to show support. Never take on the responsibility of the person's eating disorder. You cannot become the food police or bathroom patrol. Practice patience and love, but don't be manipulated.

Lastly, don't neglect your own emotional and physical health.

Binge Eating Disorder (BED) has only recently been recognized in the eating disorder field as a distinct disorder with its own set of characteristics. The criteria* for diagnosing BED are as follows:

A. Recurrent episodes of binge eating. An episode of binge eating is characterized by both of the following:
   1. eating, in a discrete period of time (e.g. within any two hour period), an amount of food that is definitely larger than most people would eat during a similar period of time in similar circumstances.
   2. a sense of lack of control over eating during the episode (e.g., a feeling that one cannot stop eating or control what or how much one is eating)

B. During most binge episodes, at least three of the following behavioral indicators of loss of control are present:
   1. eating much more rapidly than usual
   2. eating until feeling uncomfortably full
   3. eating large amounts of food when not feeling physically hungry
   4. eating alone because of being embarrassed by how much one is eating
   5. feeling disgusted with oneself, depressed, or feeling very guilty after overeating.

C. The binge eating caused marked distress

D. The binge eating occurs, on average, at least two days a week for a six-month period

E. Does not currently meet the criteria for anorexia nervosa or bulimia nervosa, purging or non-purging type.
   - from Diagnostic & Statistical Manual of Mental Disorders, American Psychiatric Assn., Fourth edition.

BED is different than bulimia nervosa in that there is no purging component, such as vomiting, laxative abuse, or excessive exercise. Most people with BED are obese. It is estimated that between 20% and 50% of all obese people suffer from BED. People with BED are more likely to have been obese as children, experienced frequent bouts of weight loss and regain, have significant body shape distortion, and have other psychiatric problems such as anxiety or depression.

Compulsive Overeating (COE) is not formally recognized as an eating disorder diagnosis. However, the term "compulsive overeating" is often used by professionals and their clients to describe a disordered eating pattern that includes repeated bouts of over eating in response to emotional triggers and an obsession with food and weight. The over eating often occurs without conscious awareness. Binge-eating, as defined in the criteria for BED, may or may not be present. Overeating is usually described as eating when not hungry, eating beyond satiety, or eating based on emotional triggers.

People with COE are not necessarily obese. Dieting is often part of this disorder and can lead to subsequent overeating, causing a dieting/overeating cycle that is repeated over and over.

Causes of BED/COE

Many factors likely contribute to the development of BED and COE. Researchers are looking into the impact of chronic dieting, sexual abuse, depression, and obsessive-compulsive disorder have on the development of these disorders.

There is great social pressure in developed countries to be thin and physically fit beyond what is necessary for maintaining good health. The ideal body size of extreme thinness and/or well-defined "ripped" muscles is unattainable for the vast majority of people. Chronically fighting the body's natural weight by undereating (dieting) has been shown to result in rebound overeating and binge-eating. Some people rebel against society's ideal body shape by overeating and under exercising. Others become so discouraged about their inability to lose weight that they give up efforts to normalize eating behavior.

Eating is a soothing behavior that leads to a sense of calmness and relaxation. When food is introduced as a way to calm down or as a reward for good behavior, one learns to self-soothe with food regardless of physical need. Overeating becomes a learned response to all manner of physical and psychological stresses, whether they be positive or negative stresses. The habit of overeating becomes so automatic that one is often not consciously aware of the behavior.

Binge eating perpetuates the overeating behavior by increasing the stomach's capacity. This, in turn, decreases the signals to the body for satiety and encourages further binge eating.

Medical and Psychological Consequences of BED/COE

Chronic binge-eating or overeating can lead to obesity. Obesity is associated with an increased risk of developing diabetes, high cholesterol, and high blood pressure. Chronic overeating and rapid eating can cause digestive problems, sleepiness, and lethargy.

People with BED or COE feel tremendous guilt about their eating behavior and shame about their body size. They tend to isolate themselves which furthers the feelings of inadequacy and the obsession with food and weight. Isolation also makes it easier to binge eat or over eat. They may have limited enjoyment and fulfillment in their lives.

The discrimination experienced by the obese is real. They suffer psychologically and financially as a result. Even obtaining good medical care may be difficult due to prejudice among physicians and other health-care providers.

Treatment Options

Most hospital-based and residential eating disorder programs treat BED along with anorexia nervosa and bulimia. Programs range from one week intensive therapy to several weeks of treatment followed by on-going out-patient treatment. Out-patient treatment is the most common treatment for COE.

Nutrition therapy and psychotherapy are combined to normalize eating/exercise behaviors and resolve underlying psychological issues. Medical monitoring for health problems associated with obesity and overeating is also incorporated. Treatment involves reconnecting one's eating to physical signals of hunger and satiety, learning healthier stress management and coping behaviors, increasing self-esteem and empowerment, reconciling unresolved family issues and traumatic events, and improving body image/acceptance. Antidepressant medication may also be included.

Self-help groups are another resource for people with BED or COE. Overeaters anonymous is available in most cities around the country and is usually advertised in the classified section of the local newspaper. Support groups are also available on the Internet.

What Loved Ones Can Do To Help

It is important to recognize that overcoming any eating disorder is extremely difficult and can take months or years of treatment, depending on the disorder's severity. Knowing about nutrition and health is not enough. One has to learn to respond to life differently. The following tips can help you be supportive.

1. Reinforce your love by being willing to listen to your loved one's struggle and give hugs when needed.
2. Do not assume weight loss will solve the problem, even if the person says it will.
3. Do not try to control the person's eating, even if you are asked to do so.
4. Ask your loved one what you can do to be most supportive, but do not accept the role of policeman over his/her food intake.
5. Let the person know you love him/her for reasons other than body size or looks.
6. Do not try to "fix" the problem by offering to go on a diet with your loved one.
7. Accept the struggle, even if you do not understand it.
8. Educate yourself about the disorder. There are many books available in bookstores or the library (see Suggested Reading List below).
9. Attend support group meetings or therapy sessions if asked to do so.
10. Model healthy eating and exercise habits. Do this as a genuine concern for your own well-being, not as a way to try and get your loved one to change.
11. Practice size acceptance of yourself, your loved one, and others. Focus on characteristics other than size or looks that you admire in yourself and others.

12. Be willing to support the recovery process. This requires allocating family funds to treatment and helping out with child rearing and other household activities when needed.
13. Recognize that it is not your job to fix your loved one. It is your job to be supportive. Tell the person about your concerns in a loving way, and offer information on resources available in the community. Then leave the rest up to her/him.

Seasonal Affective Disorder (SAD) or Winter Depression is a condition caused by a deficiency of light during winter months. SAD was identified in 1979 by Al Lewy, M.D. at OHSU who pioneered the research that is the basis of treatment protocols today. Dietitians may see clients who experience SAD, but do not know it, nor that their bingeing or weight gain is a result. SAD starts at an early age and is sometimes confused with school phobia. It affects females more than males with approximately 5% of the population having severe symptoms, and another 15% a subsyndromal version.

Some possible symptoms of SAD are:

- Increased appetite
- Binge eating of high carbohydrate foods
- Weight gain
- Increased sleep or need for sleep and difficulty waking
- Immobilized and/or suicidal ideation
- Decreased energy
- Decreased creativity

People with SAD in the Pacific Northwest begin to have difficulty in late October/early November. It is at its worst in January, and is completely improved by May or June. We can determine if a client has SAD by asking if they have noticed that their eating is increased during those months. If they have not, you can ask if they have noticed that if only during the winter months they have difficulty waking up at their usual time, or if they feel depressed or blue. If the answer is yes, and they don't experience depression at any other time of the year, suspect SAD.

SAD occurs when days are shorter because longer periods of outdoor light are not available to decrease melatonin, a hormone that causes sleepiness. Daylight (even on cloudy days) passes through the retina and signals the pineal gland to stop producing melatonin. When dawn is later, melatonin levels remain too high for wakefulness and a mood disorder resembling ordinary depression results.

SAD can be treated successfully by using special cool, bright lights of no less than 10,000 lux or light units. Avoid full spectrum as it contains ultra-violet. Most people with SAD have difficulty waking, and respond to light therapy as soon as they get up, ideally between 6 a.m.-8 a.m. They should spend 30 minutes in front of the light machine, perhaps as they eat breakfast or read the paper. They should avoid staring into the light, but rather scan across it a few times a minute for a few seconds. The closer one is to the light, the brighter, so that clients should follow the manufacturer's directions.

What is disordered eating, and how can it be prevented? Normal, healthy eating behavior may be defined as when a person eats when she or he is hungry, and stops eating when full. That is, the person is aware of and responds appropriately to hunger and satiety cues. Of course, all of us can recall a time when we have eaten past our natural fullness point, or have skipped a meal even when hungry. This does not mean everyone has disordered eating, although variations of this problem are extremely common. It is only when an individual consistently ignores feelings of hunger or fullness and this pattern of behavior becomes usual for them that the person may be said to have disordered eating. "Disordered eating" covers a broad spectrum of eating behavior including eating disorders, while the term "eating disorder" is defined quite specifically by diagnostic criteria.

Some possible causes of disordered eating include negative body image, low self-esteem, peer pressure, and lack of information about how eating and dieting can affect health. In order to prevent these problems, we must look at what is believed to cause them. Both of the topics mentioned above note that eating disorders fill a need for the individual. For example, eating is a self-soothing activity. It is quite possible that a "cause" of overeating might be that the child has not learned any other way to soothe himself or calm down when he is upset. Similarly, a teen girl might find her need for attention met when she loses weight after being on a diet. Like all dysfunctions, the principle of "overdetermination" applies. There are many causes and predisposing factors, which in combination can influence a person to adopt a disordered eating pattern. Some would say that just being a member (especially female) of western society, is a predisposing factor. Foreyt and Goodrick in their book "Living Without Dieting" point out that western culture is a "lookist" culture, overemphasizing appearance and underemphasizing human qualities. Lookism, like racism or sexism, defines people by external characteristics that have nothing to do with a person's real abilities. Most young people are strongly influenced by media images which associate unrealistic thinness with beauty, sexiness, money, power and happiness. Lookism is not talked about, but is a very real social force.

Recent research shows that body dissatisfaction is the single strongest predictor of eating disorder symptcmolgy (Phelps, Johnston and Augustyniak, 1999)*. Helping teen girls (and boys) recognize the positive attributes of their physical appearance may be the most effective prevention strategy we have. This approach increases feelings of self-efficacy, helping them feel "OK". It also helps reduce the internalization of the unnatural "ideal" body standard, and lets them realize that each person expresses their own inner beauty differently. It is important to understand that young people are bombarded with hundreds of messages about attractiveness every day. All influential adults play a role in letting kids know what is "right" with their looks. Adults who are not comfortable with their own appearance may be most hard pressed to send positive messages to teens.

Girls and women are more at risk than boys and men, probably due to unreasonable expectations for female body shape and distorted expressions of female beauty portrayed in the media. Debra Waterhouse's excellent book "Like Mother Like Daughter" traces the legacy of dieting and disordered eating through the generations, while offering strategies to break this destructive cycle.

Boys and men are not exempt from the pressures to modify their bodies. Unfortunately, exploitation of men based on appearance is on the increase, and this is likely to result in greater numbers of males with disordered eating. Magazines covers of men with abdominal muscle definition few can ever achieve are found in every check out stand, next to the women's magazines featuring impossibly thin but full busted female models. Young people view these pictures as the standard of attractiveness and try hard to measure up.

Sports can have a mixed effect on body image as well. Studies show that girls who participate in sports have higher scores for self esteem and are less likely to be victimized by others. However, it is well known that certain sports which emphasize thinness, like gymnastics, dance and figure skating, put girls at higher risk. For boys, wrestling can contribute to dysfunctional eating behaviors and purging in order to attain/maintain an unnatural weight. Parents and coaches need to give healthy, non-diet messages to teen athletes. Coaches especially have a strong influence on whether an athlete learns to be their best with the body shape and size they have, or ends up wasting precious mental and physical energy on artificial weight goals. Dieting has a negative impact on sports performance. Good sports nutrition, on the other hand, can enhance performance on and off the playing field.

Prevention Strategies

Parents, teachers and coaches: Your example matters! Practice healthy eating behaviors. Eat when you get up in the morning, and eat every 4 hours or so throughout the day. This will help your body get on schedule, so that you will experience hunger on a regular basis. Stop eating when you are full! Your body knows better than you do how to maintain a healthy weight.

Coaches: Your actions and your words are more important than you know! Many cases of eating disorders in athletes start when coaches tell them that weight loss will improve performance. Read up on sports nutrition. Consider getting a registered dietitian to speak to team members and parents.

Mothers: Be aware of your own weight issues. Dieting is not "normal", despite what media influences may say. If your teen is experiencing difficulties, don't blame yourself. Instead, be part of the solution by treating your own body with respect.

All influential adults: Listen to what you say! Our language has incorporated many myths that you may spread unconsciously. Were you "good" today by eating salad, but "bad" yesterday when you ate a brownie? There are no good and bad foods. All foods can fit into a healthy diet. Talk to kids about what really is good and bad, and share your values with them.

Help children learn how to get their needs met. Teach them how to ask for what they need. Many experts believe that disordered eating behaviors are a language used by people who don't have the words to say "that makes me mad" or "I feel hurt."

Make a point of recognizing kids' attractive physical features. Many times we spoil a compliment by adding "if you didn't have such heavy legs" or some such negative remark. Praise really won't spoil kids, even when it comes to appearance! Criticism will not help them lose weight, it will only damage their self esteem.

Teach critical thinking skills. Help kids think problems through. Does it really make sense to think that going on a diet will solve the problem?

Avoid "horror" stories of anorexia or bulimia. Scaring kids usually doesn't work and may teach dysfunctional behavior.

Help children relax. If relaxation means sitting in front of the TV eating chips, the child is being set up for a weight problem as well as missing out on skills needed to reduce stress. Use physical activity as a stress release. You know it's working if you can say you had fun!

Exercise in moderation. Physical activity is for fun and health, not to burn calories or achieve a certain percent body fat.

Examine cultural values. Do you really think its necessary to look a certain way in order to be happy? Promote size acceptance as part of the natural diversity of human beings.

Accept your own body. It is just as hard for adults to resist negative media messages as it is for kids, especially since we've been hearing them longer! Helping kids can be a reason to help ourselves.

Develop "learned hardiness". Kids can learn to roll with the punches and resist influences that depress or discourage them. Encourage activities that build character.

Avoid dieting! Research shows that most eating disorders started with a diet. Diets don't work! See the resource list below for weight management strategies that do work.

Individuals who exercise compulsively can be diagnosed as having either anorexia or non-purging type bulimia. Compulsive exercisers use activity to "purge" the body of excess calories in order to maintain abnormal eating patterns or to prevent weight gain that approaches normal weight. Because athletes and athleticism are so highly regarded in our culture, it's particularly difficult to convince someone engaged in this compulsion that it is actually an illness. Social acceptance of exercise helps those with this disorder maintain the illusion of good health, even a feeling of superiority, as they hide in their illness.

The question is then, when is exercise compulsive?

Signs and Symptoms of Exercise Bulimia adapted from the organization Anorexia Nervosa and Related Eating Disorders.

The individual may:

- often choose to exercise beyond the requirements for good health
- be fanatic about their weight and diet
- steal time from work, school, relationships, and social gatherings to exercise
- focus only on the challenge and forget that exercise can be fun
- define self worth in terms of performance
- rarely or never be satisfied with athletic achievements
- be unable to savor victory; always pushing on to the next challenge
- justify excessive behavior by defining self as a "special" elite athlete
- use exercise compulsively to control weight
- experience strong feelings of guilt or anxiety if unable to exercise
- not allow time off to heal injuries
- hide from emotional pain by working out

- cause comment from friends and family about the amount of time engaged in physical activity.

Consequences

There are physical and psychological consequences to overexercising; some are listed below:

Physical:

- Stress fractures
- Tendinitis
- Damaged bones, joints, tendons and ligaments
- Irregular menstruation
- Osteoporosis
- Amenorrhea
- Chronic Fatigue Syndrome
- Malnutrition
- Anemia
- Dehydration
- Fatigue
- Insomnia Psychological:
- Obsessive thoughts
- Compulsive behaviors
- Self worth measured only in terms of performance
- Abandoned relationships
- Damaged careers
- Lower grades in school
- Depression
- Anxiety
- Social isolation

How do I know if I have a problem with compulsive exercise? You can take this quiz by answering yes or no to the questions below to see if you may have a problem with overexercising.

1. Do you find that you regularly adjust your exercise according to how much you ate earlier or on the preceding day?
2. Are you concerned to terrified about being overweight?
3. Did your interest in exercise begin with a desire to lose weight?
4. Do you fear not exercising each day because you think you'll gain weight?

5. Are you preoccupied with food and calories and calculate what you are allowed to eat each day according to how much time you can give to exercise?
6. Have you gone on eating binges where you feel you cannot stop?
7. Do you exercise an excessive amount after a binge?
8. Are you preoccupied with being thinner, and have a lower body mass/lean muscle ratio as elite athletes do?
9. Do you think about burning calories as you exercise?
10. Do you ever vomit, take laxatives, or diuretics after a meal or binge to feel thinner or to attempt to lose calories?
11. Do you feel virtuous when dieting, restricting your dietary intake, or exercising?
12. Do others tell you that you exercise too much?

If you can answer yes to six or more of these questions, your exercise behavior may be based in an eating disorder.

Dealing With Mid-Life Weight Issues

A Case Study on Perimenopausal Weight Gain

An active, 45 year old woman decides to try meeting with a Registered Dietitian to help her lose weight. She is 5 feet 4 inches tall and weighs 165 pounds, the most she has ever weighed in her entire life. The woman's name is Mary.

Mary reports that she has been dieting her entire adult life to maintain a weight of 120 pounds, the weight that she should weigh according to the insurance industry charts. She watches her diet very carefully, eating mostly low fat foods and consuming around 1200 calories per day. Mary has never had to exercise to keep her weight down—dieting has always worked except for when she would go through phases of binge eating followed by weight gain. She says she was always too tired to exercise. She admits to yo yoing up and down 20 pounds with her weight over the years, and states that after having her second child at age 35 dieting stopped working. During the past 5 years, Mary has gradually gained 20 pounds even though she has watched her diet very carefully and most of the time does not eat many "bad foods." Mary is very frustrated with her weight, and she wants to know if starting a high protein, low carbohydrate diet is the way to go.

The Registered Dietitian recommends the following to Mary:

1. During the perimenopausal period (ages 35-55 for most women), the female fat cell actually grows larger in response to declining production of estrogen. This results in an increase in body fat, particularly in the abdominal area. There is a good reason for this to occur. After menopause is when women are at the highest risk for osteoporosis. The body works to combat this by preferentially storing estrogen in fat cells in the abdominal area, where the estrogen is easily accessible to help keep calcium in the bones. An increase in body fat during this time is normal and healthy for the body. It is unrealistic for most peri or postmenopausal women to have less than 30% body fat.
2. Many women who have chronically dieted experience a large weight gain during this time. Chronic dieting is usually a sign that the person is keeping her weight artificially low, or at less than her set-point body weight (the weight your body is genetically programmed to weigh). The more dieting a woman does, the more fat the body stores to protect itself. Weight charts are really not a good indicator of set-point weight, as set-point weight is very individual and is believed to be genetically determined. A woman's set-point weight is the weight where she can eat all foods moderately in response to her body's hunger and fullness signals, along with regular, moderate exercise.
3. Exercise is the key to weight management at any age, especially in mid-life. Many women have substituted chronic dieting in place of exercise, resulting in a loss of muscle and bone and an increase in body fat. After obtaining approval from your physician, begin a program of walking, biking, swimming, dancing or some other activity for 20 minutes 3 days per week. The key is to pick an activity that is fun for you, and preferably something you can do with a partner. Women who exercise with a friend or spouse are more likely to maintain their program on a long-term basis. After a week or so at 20 minutes, increase your time spent exercising to 30 minutes, and then gradually over time increase to 45 minutes to one hour. The reality is that in order to lose the weight and reach your set-point body weight, you will need to do about 5 hours of

aerobic exercise per week. Most perimenopausal women maintain a healthy weight by doing an activity they enjoy for 3-5 hours per week.

4. There are no "good" or "bad" foods. All foods have nutritional value, and depriving yourself can lead to binging. Work on eating in response to your body's hunger and fullness signals, instead of external triggers like stress, boredom, or a structured diet plan. If you eat when you are hungry and stop when you are full, your body will move towards its set-point weight. High protein, low carbohydrate diets are unbalanced nutritionally and tend to cause fatigue, cravings for sugar and bread, and depression in susceptible people. You need a diet high in complex carbohydrates to provide energy and allow for fat burning during exercise.
5. All perimenopausal women need to accept that their bodies will not look the same as when they were 20 years old. Work on appreciating and accepting your natural body type. Healthy, moderate eating and exercise will help you to be happier and more productive during the peri and postmenopausal years.

Almost a decade ago doctors and coaches began to notice a trend in female athletes to enhance their athletic performance by achieving very low body weights. They also noticed that these women athletes were engaging in potentially harmful methods of weight control and that many suffered from amenorrhea and bone loss. In 1992, the American College of Sports Medicine named the collection of symptoms seen in this population as "The Female Athlete Triad". The triad is especially prevalent in sports that emphasize the aesthetic of leanness such as gymnastics, figure skating, diving and dance. It is also seen in sports such as swimming and running, where leanness is thought to help gain the competitive edge. While the triad is most common in women participating in these sports, it can affect any athlete.

Determining the prevalence rate of the triad is difficult. Most of the data is equivocal. There are a number of methodological weaknesses in most of the studies due to either self-developed questionnaires, lack of control groups, and/or comparison difficulties due to the different measures used. These studies use different definitions for amenorrhea and disordered eating which further skews results. Evidence suggests that the syndrome is quite common. While the prevalence rate of disordered eating among non-athletes is thought to be between 3 and 8 percent, disordered eating and amenorrhea are thought to affect anywhere for 15 to 62 percent of female athletes.

The female athlete triad is a serious syndrome consisting of three separate but interrelated components: disordered eating, amenorrhea, and osteoporosis. Disordered eating affects theses athletes by causing decreased energy intake, decreased nutrient intake, decreased resting metabolic rate, low body fat stores, gastrointestinal problems (constipation, diarrhea, reflux, bloating, and post prandial distress) hypothermia, menstrual disturbances or delayed puberty, and increased risk of anorexia, bulimia, osteoporosis, morbidity and mortality. The triad increases the incidence of osteopenia, bone injury, stress fractures, and scoliosis. There is also a marked increase in psychological stress with increased difficulty handling the stress of competition, which can lead to decreased physical performance. What many coaches and athletes don't seem to understand is that this quest for sharp reductions in body fat in the hopes of gaining the competitive edge has both long and short-term consequences for woman's health.

Disordered Eating

In an effort to lose more body fat, an athlete may begin to consume less energy than is necessary for his/her activity level. She can fall into a pattern of restrictive eating that lead to believing that once normal portions of food are now too much. Or she becomes phobic of many foods that were once enjoyed and avoid them believing that the food will cause weight gain. Vegetarianism is commonly adopted to further curtail and assert control over calorie and fat intake, as the rules of vegetarianism further enhance restrictive eating practices. Over time the list of acceptable foods become shorter and variety may be diminished to only two or three foods. If continued for too long these individuals can develop a full-blown eating disorder.

Athletes have been known to use many compensatory mechanisms for achieving a desired weight such as abusing diuretics, laxatives and engaging in self-induced vomiting.

While these activities were once overlooked as required behavior to achieve the competitive advantage, today we know the consequences of these eating disordered behaviors upon one's physical and emotional health. These once acceptable weight loss tactics should be addressed with professionals once they are discovered.

It may be that sports, especially those in which the disorder is most prevalent, attracts those with eating disorders. Sport competition attracts those who are highly focused, motivated and perfectionistic. These are the primary personality traits of disordered eaters and may have many of them using their sport to legitimize their eating disorder. It is difficult to see that there is a problem when the patient is excelling at her sport. In these cases the illness just looks like the quirky or superstitious behavior of an elite athlete. Often eating disorders can go on for years without affecting performance. It is not until many years later that the nutrient and energy imbalance, which produces subtle changes in physiology and psychology, begin to take their toll.

Amenorrhea

There is a relationship between menstrual disturbances, level of athletic training and disordered eating; but how they are connected is not completely understood. Many believe it begins with the restricting of caloric intake coupled with rigorous exercise leading to decreased fat stores, which then decreases the body's ability to produce hormones necessary for the reproductive cycle to continue normally. It was once thought that 12% body fat was the lowest percent a woman could obtain and still have good health. It is now known at this level a woman would be putting her health in danger. It is when female body fat percentages plunge below approximately 17%, that amenorrhea begins. It is thought that as women decrease caloric intake and increase energy output through excessive athletic training schedules, the body goes into a state of energy imbalance of famine. The body responds by shutting off activity that isn't essential to life. The first system to go is the reproductive system. During a prolonged energy deficit, the body shuts down the ovarian production of estrogen. It is thought that body wisdom understands that in the famine mode there is not enough energy to sustain new life and menses ceases.

Unfortunately, many doctors and coaches believe that amenorrhea is a sign of athleticism. They believe that it is a natural side effect to training. Amenorrhea is the cessation of menses for at least three consecutive months. Any athlete exhibiting amenorrhea should be questioned for disordered eating.

Osteoporosis

The third side effect, low bone density, may be the most dangerous part of the triad due to its irreversibility and its effect on the long-term health of these women. It is believed that the lack of estrogen due to secondary amenorrhea decreases bone density. An early sign of bone loss is stress fracture. This diagnosis can be elusive because it often doesn't show up in a x-ray. Since bone development is believed to occur only up to the age of thirty, adolescence and young adulthood is a prime time for the beginning of osteoporosis. Studies show that amenorrheic athletes have a lower bone mineral density that those with regular menstrual cycles, increasing their risk of osteoporosis. These women may be at greater risk for hip or vertebral spine compression fractures, which can be very painful and debilitating.

Understanding the female athlete triad, the importance of proper nutrition and a positive body image is imperative for coaches, trainers, parents and athletes. The following suggestions for coaches and trainers can also help:

- Avoid weighing athletes and obtaining body composition data.
- Observe meals to check for disordered eating patterns.
- Encourage a snack period midway through practice to replenish energy.

CHAPTER 6

ATHLETES & NUTRITION

Pre-Game & Post-Game Advice

The following information provides you with a quick look at what works

best in nutritional care for the athlete. For more information you may want to consult a registered dietitian.

The goals of nutritional care for athletes are simple and straightforward. For the most part, nutritional care should:

- ensure that athletes have adequate fluids during periods of active training and competition
- provide adequate calories to meet growth and development needs (if in youth and adolescent years)
- provide calories to meet extra needs of physical activity
- supply nutrients from food
- instill sound nutrition principles and practices that will last a lifetime

The best eating habits for the athlete may be as follows:

1. Design a meal pattern that fits your daily routine. Plan to eat at least three times a day. Use snacks between regular meals to help meet caloric and nutrient needs.
2. Eat a diet rich in complex carbohydrates (starches). Starchy foods such as pasta, breads, cereals, potatoes, corn, peas and others provide a major energy source to fuel your activities. These foods are also a source of fiber, vitamins, and minerals.
3. Drink sufficient fluids to stay hydrated during training and competition periods - don't wait until you are thirsty to drink.
4. Eat a diet that contains a variety of foods from breads and cereals; fruits; vegetables; meat and meat substitutes, and dairy groups. It is your best insurance for getting needed nutrients.

PRE-GAME RULES

1. Eat lightly before an athletic competition.
2. Eat complex carbohydrates, keep protein and fat intakes low since these slow digestion.
3. Avoid bulky foods. They may stimulate bowel movements. Bulky foods include raw fruits and vegetables, dry beans and peas, popcorn.
4. Avoid gas-forming foods such as vegetables from the cabbage family and cooked dry beans
5. Eat slowly and chew well.
6. Drink water to be adequately hydrated. One suggestion is to drink 2 ½ cups water 1 to 2 hours before the event. Follow this by drinking about 1 ¼ cups water 15 minutes before the event.
7. Avoid drastic changes in your normal diet routine immediately prior to competition. Some athletes prefer to use favorite foods which may give them a psychological edge.

POST-GAME RULES

1. Eat carbohydrate-rich foods and beverages as soon as possible after competition. They will replenish glycogen stores quickly and get the athlete back into performance shape. Fruits, juices, high carbohydrate drinks, pop are examples.
2. Replace fluids that have been lost. For every pound that is lost, drink 2 cups of fluids.
3. Replace any potassium or sodium that has been lost during competition or training by using foods. Fruits and vegetables are excellent sources of potassium. Replace sodium by eating salty foods.
4. Return to your normal high carbohydrate diet at your next meal.

CLARIFICATION ABOUT SPORTS NUTRITION

BEST DIET FOR AN ATHLETE

It's important that an athlete's diet provides the right amount of energy, the 50-plus nutrients the body needs and adequate water. No single food or supplement can do this. A variety of foods are needed every day. But, just as there is more than one way to achieve a goal, there is more than one way to follow a nutritious diet.

NUTRITIONAL NEEDS OF ATHLETES & FROM NONATHLETES

Competitive athletes, sedentary individuals and people who exercise for health and fitness all need the same nutrients. However, because of the intensity of their sport or training program, some athletes have higher calorie and fluid requirements. Eating a variety of foods to meet increased calorie needs helps to ensure that the athletes diet contains appropriate amounts of carbohydrate, protein, vitamins and minerals.

DIETARY GUIDELINES TO ATHLETES

Health and nutrition professionals recommend that 55-60% of the calories in our diet come from carbohydrate, no more than 30% from fat and the remaining 10-15% from protein. While the exact percentages may vary slightly for some athletes based on their sport or training program, these guidelines will promote health and serve as the basis for a diet that will maximize performance.

DAILY NEED OF CALORIES

This depends on your age, body size, sport and training program. For example, a 250-pound weight lifter needs for calories than a 98-pound gymnast. Exercise or training may increase calorie needs by as much as 1,000 to 1,500 calories a day.

The best way to determine if you're getting too few or too many calories is to monitor your weight. Keeping within your ideal competitive weight range means that you are getting the right amount of calories.

BETTER REPLACING FLUIDS-WATER OR SPORTS DRINKS

Depending on how muscular you are, 55-70% of your body weight is water. Being "hydrated" means maintaining your body's fluid level. When you sweat, you lose water which must be replaced if you want to perform your best. You need to drink fluids before, during and after all workouts and events.

Whether you drink water or a sports drink is a matter of choice. However, if your workout or event lasts for more than 90 minutes, you may benefit from the carbohydrates provided by sports drinks. A sports drink that contains 15-18 grams of carbohydrate in every 8 ounces of fluid should be used. Drinks with a higher carbohydrate content will delay the absorption of water and may cause dehydration, cramps, nausea or diarrhea. There are a variety of sports drinks on the market. Be sure to experiment with sports drinks during practice instead of trying them for the first time the day of an event.

ELECTROLYTES

Electrolytes are nutrients that affect fluid balance in the body and are necessary for our nerves and muscles to function. Sodium and potassium are the two electrolytes most often added to sports drinks. Generally, electrolyte replacement is not needed during short bursts of exercise since sweat is approximately 99% water and less than 1% electrolytes. Water, in combination with a well-balanced diet, will restore normal fluid and electrolyte levels in the body. However, replacing electrolytes may be beneficial during continuous activity of longer than 2 hours, especially in a hot environment.

ENERGY NEEDED BY MUSCLES DURING EXERCISE

Most activities use a combination of fat and carbohydrate as energy sources. How hard and how long you work out, your level of fitness and your diet will affect the type of fuel your body uses. For short-term high-intensity activities like sprinting, athletes rely mostly on carbohydrate for energy. During low-intensity exercises like walking, the body uses more fat for energy.

CARBOHYDRATES

Carbohydrates are sugar and starches found in foods like breads, cereals, fruits, vegetables, pasta, milk, honey, syrups and table sugar. Carbohydrates are the preferred source of energy for your body. Regardless of origin, your body breaks down carbohydrates into glucose that your blood carries to cells to be used for energy. Carbohydrates provide 4 calories per gram, while fat provides 9 calories per gram. Your body cannot differentiate between glucose that comes from starches or sugars. Glucose from either source provides energy for working muscles.

ATHLETES SHOULD EAT A LOT OF CARBOHYDRATES

When you are training or competing, your muscles need energy to perform. One source of energy for working muscles is glycogen which is made from carbohydrates and stored in your muscles. Every time you work out, you use some of your glycogen. If you don't consume enough carbohydrates, your glycogen stores become depleted, which can result in fatigue. Both sugars and starches are effective in replenishing glycogen stores.

WHEN AND WHAT TO EAT BEFORE COMPETION

Performance depends largely on the foods consumed during the days and weeks leading up to an event. If you regularly eat a varied, carbohydrate-rich diet you are in good standing and probably have ample glycogen stores to fuel activity. The purpose of the precompetition meal is to prevent hunger and to provide the water and additional energy the athlete will need during competition. Most athletes eat 2 to 4 hours before their event. However, some athletes perform their best if they eat a small amount 30 minutes before competing, while others eat nothing for 6 hours beforehand.

For many athletes, carbohydrate-rich foods serve as the basis of the meal. However, there is no magic pre-event diet. Simply choose foods and beverages that you enjoy and that don't bother your stomach. Experiment during the weeks before an event to see which foods work best for you.

EATING SUGARY FOODS

In the past, athletes were warned that eating sugary foods before exercise could hurt performance by causing a drop in blood glucose levels. Recent studies, however, have shown that consuming sugar up to 30 minutes before an event does not diminish performance. In fact, evidence suggests that a sugar-containing precompetition beverage or snack may improve performance during endurance workouts and events.

WHAT IS CARBOHYDRATE LOADING?

Carbohydrate loading is a technique used to increase the amount of glycogen in muscles. For five to seven days before an event, the athlete eats 10-12 grams of carbohydrate per kilogram body weight and gradually reduces the intensity of the workouts. (To find out how much you weigh in kilograms, simply divide your weight in pounds by 2.2.) The day before the event, the athlete rests and eats the same high-carbohydrate diet. Although carbohydrate loading may be beneficial for athletes participating in endurance sports which require 90 minutes or more of non-stop effort, most athletes needn't worry about carbohydrate loading. Simply eating a diet that derives more than half of its calories from carbohydrates will do.

NEED OF EXTRA VITAMINS AND MINERALS

Athletes need to eat about 1,800 calories a day to get the vitamins and minerals they need for good health and optimal performance. Since most athletes eat more than this amount, vitamin and mineral supplements are needed only in special situations. Athletes who follow vegetarian diets or who avoid an entire group of foods (for example, never drink milk) may need a supplement to make up for the vitamins and minerals not being supplied by food. A multivitamin-mineral pill that supplies 100% of the

Recommended Dietary Allowance (RDA) will provide the nutrients needed. An athlete who frequently cuts back on calories, especially below the 1,800 calorie level, is not only at risk for inadequate vitamin and mineral intake, but also may not be getting enough carbohydrate. Since vitamins and minerals do not provide energy, they cannot replace the energy provided by carbohydrates.

WILL EXTRA PROTEIN HELP BUILD MUSCLE MASS?

Many athletes, especially those on strength-training programs or who participate in power sports, are told that eating a ton of protein or taking protein supplements will help them gain muscle weight. However, the true secret to building muscle is training hard and consuming enough calories. While some extra protein is needed to build muscle, most American diets provide more than enough protein. Between 1.0 and 1.5 grams of protein per kilogram body weight per day is sufficient if your calorie intake is adequate and you're eating a variety of foods. For a 150-pound athlete, that represents 68-102 grams of protein a day.

IMPORTANCE OF IRON

Hemoglobin, which contains iron, is the part of red blood cells that carries oxygen from the lungs to all parts of the body, including muscles. Since your muscles need oxygen to produce energy, if you have low iron levels in your blood, you may tire quickly. Symptoms of iron deficiency include fatigue, irritability, dizziness, headaches and lack of appetite. Many times, however, there are no symtoms at all. A blood test is the best way to find out if your iron level is low. It is recommended that athletes have their hemoglobin level checked once a year.

The RDA for iron is 15 milligrams a day for women and 10 milligrams a day for men. Red meat is the richest source of iron, but fish and poultry also are good sources. Fortified breakfast cereals, beans and green leafy vegetables also contain iron. Our bodies absorb the iron found in animal products best.

IRON SUPPLEMENT

Taking iron supplements will not improve performance unless an athlete is truly iron deficient. Too much iron can cause constipation, diarrhea, nausea and may interfere with the absorption of other nutrients such as cooper and zinc. Therefore, iron supplements should not be taken without proper medical supervision.

IMPORTANCE OF CALCIUM

Calcium is needed for strong bones and proper muscle function. Dairy foods are the best source of calcium. However, studies show that many female athletes who are trying to lose weight cut back on dairy products. Female athletes who don't get enough calcium may be at risk for stress fractures and, when they're older, osteoporosis. Young women between the ages of 9 and 18 need about 1,300 milligrams of calcium a day. Adults aged 19 through 50 need 1,000 milligrams daily, while those 51 and older should aim for 1,200 milligrams. Low-fat dairy products are a rich source of calcium and also are low in fat and calories.

The following table of popular foods includes foods rich in carbohydrates (CHO), protein, iron and/or calcium. The nutrient analysis for each food was obtained using The Food Processor II computer program.

Nutrient Content of Selected Foods

Nutrient Content of Selected Foods							
Food	Serving Size	Energy (kcal)	Protein (g)	CHO (g)	Fat (g)	Calcium (mg)	Iron (mg)
Lean Beef	3 ounces	189	27	0	8	4	2.9
Hamburger	3 ounces	246	20	0	18	9	2.1
Lean Pork, Broiled	3 ounces	196	27	0	9	4	.8
Chicken, Breast	3 ounces	167	25	0	7	12	.9
Egg, Hard-Boiled	1 whole	77	6	1	5	25	.6
Peanut Butter	2 tablespoons	190	8	7	16	11	.5
Roasted Peanuts	1 ounce	164	7	5	14	24	.5
Navy Beans, Cooked	1/2 cup	129	8	24	0	64	2.2
Salmon, Broiled/Baked	3 ounces	183	23	0	9	6	.5
Salmon, Canned With Bones	3 ounces	118	17	0	5	182	.7
Milk, Whole	1 cup	150	8	11	8	291	.1
2% Low-Fat	1 cup	121	8	12	5	297	.1
1% Low-Fat	1 cup	102	8	12	3	300	.1
Skim	1 cup	85	8	12	0	302	.1
Yogurt, Low-Fat	1 cup	193	11	31	3	388	.2
Cheddar Cheese	1.5 ounces	171	11	0	14	305	.3
Cottage Cheese, 2%	1/2 cup	102	16	4	2	78	.2
Ice Cream, Vanilla	1/2 cup	134	2	16	7	88	.1
Bread, White/ Wheat	1 slice	72	3	13	1	35	1.0
Bran Flakes, Fortified	1 ounce	91	4	25	0	14	8.1
Muffin, Bran	1 whole	125	3	19	6	60	1.4
Cookie, Choc. Chip	3 whole	139	2	19	6	6	.8
Baked Potato	1 whole	220	5	51	0	20	2.8
Spaghetti	1/2 cup	98	3	20	0	5	1.0
Green Peas	1/2 cup	63	4	11	0	19	1.2
Broccoli, Cooked	1/2 cup	22	2	4	0	36	.7
Banana	1 whole	105	1	28	0	7	.1
Orange	1 whole	60	1	15	0	52	.1
Butter	1 tablespoon	102	0	0	12	3	0
Margarine	1 tablespoon	102	0	0	11	4	0
Table Sugar	1 teaspoon	16	0	4	0	0	0
Jelly	1 teaspoon	16	0	4	0	1	0

CHAPTER 7

DIET PLAN FOR EVERY AGE GROUP

Toddler's Diet

You'll probably notice a sharp drop in your toddler's appetite after his first birthday. Suddenly he's picky about what he eats, turns his head away after just a few bites, or resists coming to the table at mealtimes. It may seem as if he should be eating more now that he's so active, but there's a good reason for the change. His growth rate has slowed, and he really doesn't require as much food now.

Your toddler needs about 1,000 calories a day to meet his needs for growth, energy, and good nutrition. If you've ever been on a 1,000-calorie diet, you know it's not a lot of food. But your child will do just fine with it, divided among three small meals and two snacks a day. Don't count on his always eating it that way; however, because the eating habits of toddlers are erratic and unpredictable from one day to the next. He may eat everything in sight at breakfast but almost nothing else for the rest of the day. Or he may eat only his favorite food for three days in a row, then reject it entirely. Your toddler needs foods from the same four basic nutrition groups that you do:

Meat, fish, poultry eggs, Dairy products
Fruits and vegetables
Cereal grains, potatoes
Rice, breads, pasta

When planning your child's menu, remember that cholesterol and other fats are very important for his normal growth and development, so they should not be restricted during this period.

By his first birthday, your child should be able to handle most of the foods you serve the rest of the family but with a few precautions. Be sure the food is cool enough so that it won't burn his mouth. Test the temperature yourself, because he'll dig in without considering the heat. Try to avoid foods that are heavily spiced, salted, buttered, or sweetened. These additions prevent your child from experiencing the natural taste of foods, and they may be harmful to his long-term good health. Young children seem to be more sensitive than adults to these flavorings, and may reject heavily spiced foods.

Your little one can still choke on chunks of food that are hard and large enough to plug his airway, so make sure anything you given him is mashed or cut into small, easily chewable pieces. Never offer him peanuts, grapes, carrots, whole or large sections of hot dogs, meat sticks, or hard candies. Hot dogs and carrots in particular should be quartered lengthwise and then sliced into small pieces. Also, make sure your toddler eats only while seated and supervised by an adult. "Eating on the run" increases his risk of choking. By his first birthday or soon thereafter, your toddler should drink his liquids from a cup. He'll need less milk now, because he'll get most of his calories from solid foods.

To get a better understanding of what an average day's meals should look like, take a look at the sample menu below:

Sample One Day Menu

This menu is planned for a one-year-old child who weighs approximately 21 pounds.

1 tablespoon = ½ ounce (15 cc)
1 teaspoon = 1/3 tablespoon (5 cc)
1 cup = 8 ounces (240 cc)

BREAKFAST

½ cup iron-fortified breakfast cereal or 1 cooked egg (not more than 3 eggs per week)

¼ cup whole milk (with cereal)
½ cup juice
Add to cereal one of the following:

½ banana, sliced
2-3 large sliced strawberries

SNACK

1 slice toast or whole wheat muffin

1-2 tablespoons cream cheese or peanut butter (spread)
1 cup whole milk

LUNCH

½ sandwich-tuna, egg salad, peanut butter, or cold cuts
½ cup cooked green vegetables
½ cup juice

SNACK

1-2 ounces cubed cheese, or 2-3 tablespoons pitted and diced dates

1 cup whole milk

DINNER

2-3 ounces cooked meat, ground or diced
½ cup cooked yellow or orange vegetables
½ cup pasta, rice, or potato
½ cup whole milk

Healthy Food Choices: 2 to 5 Years

The following suggestions for healthy food choices are based on the Dietary Guidelines for Americans, developed through research by the US Department of Health and Human Services and the US Department of Agriculture. The number of servings and serving sizes are intended for children between 2 and 5 years old. When a range is given for a serving size, the smaller portion is generally appropriate for a 2 or 3 year old, while the larger portion is appropriate for a 4 or 5 year old.

Breads, cereals, rice, and pasta (4-5 or more servings)

Examples of servings:

½ - 1 slice whole-grain bread
½ bagel
½ - ¾ cup unsweetened breakfast cereal
¼ - ½ cup cooked pasta or rice
2-5 whole-grain crackers
Other good choices: cornbread, English muffins, muffins, rice cakes

Vegetables (2 or more servings)

Examples of servings:

¼ - ½ cup cooked vegetables
1/3 - ½ cup raw vegetables
Good choices: asparagus, beets, broccoli, carrots, cauliflower, corn, green and red peppers, green beans, kale, peas, potato, pumpkin, squash, sweet potato, tomato, vegetable juices, zucchini

Fruit (2 or more servings)

Examples of servings:

¼ - 1 piece of fruit
¼ - ½ cup cooked fruit
½ cup juice
Good choices: apples, applesauce, apricots, bananas, cantaloupe, fruit cocktail, 100% fruit juices, grapefruit, kiwifruit, nectarines, oranges, peaches, plums, strawberries, watermelon

Dairy products (3-4 servings)

Examples of servings:

¾ cup milk
½ - ¾ ounce low-fat cheese
½ - ¾ cup low-fat yogurt
Other good choices: low-fat cottage cheese, custard, ice milk

Meat, fish, poultry, and legumes (2 or 3 servings)

Examples of servings:

1-2 ounces lean meat, fish, poultry, or tofu
1 egg
¼ cup cooked dried beans
1-2 tbsp peanut butter
Other good choices: shellfish, dried peas, lentils, reduced-fat cold cuts

Facts on Fat

Children younger than age 2 need as much as 50% of their daily calories from fat for healthy growth and brain development. After age 2, up to 30% of calories should be derived from fat. Once your child is 2 or 3 years old, you can start reducing dietary fat by:

- switching from whole milk to low-fat or nonfat milk
- serving more fish and poultry and cutting back on red meat
- removing the skin from poultry and trimming fat from meats
- reducing butter and margarine use
- using low-fat cooking methods such as baking, broiling, grilling, poaching, and steaming
- serving fiber-rich foods, including whole-grain breads, cereals, dried peas and beans, fruits, and vegetables

Facts on Fiber

Fiber becomes important in your child's diet after age 3. Dietary fiber may play a role in reducing the chances of heart disease and cancer later in life. If you follow the suggestions on fruit and vegetables servings each day, and you make sure to buy only whole-grain breads and cereals, you'll be well on the way toward helping your child develop good eating habits he'll continue through his life.

You can boost fiber by serving fresh salad with your meals, adding oat or wheat bran to any baked goods you make, and offering legumes such as chickpeas, lentils, and kidney beans at least once a week. If you think that your child isn't getting much fiber, be sure to increase his fiber intake gradually, since excessive fiber can cause painful bloating and gas. Don't forget to have kids drink plenty of water each day as well, since liquid intake can help reduce the chances of fiber-related intestinal distress. Be aware that excessive fiber intake can interfere with the body's absorption of crucial vitamins and minerals.

Calcium Counts

Making sure your toddler or preschooler gets enough calcium should be another priority. Sufficient calcium now can mean stronger, healthier bones for your child later. Children ages 1 to 3 require 500 milligrams of calcium each day; from age 4 to age 8, the requirement is 800 milligrams each day. After age 8, the requirement jumps to 1,300 milligrams per day. You can meet these guidelines by offering your children good sources of calcium such as:

- low-fat or nonfat milk
- low-fat or nonfat yogurt
- low-fat cheese
- tofu
- salmon (with bones)
- calcium-fortified fruit juices
- ice cream (occasionally)

Taming the Sweet Tooth

Almost everyone has a sweet tooth, and that attraction to sweets can make it difficult to keep toddlers and preschoolers from choosing candy, cookies, and cakes over healthier fare. You can't do much to take the sweet tooth out of the kid, but you can keep sweets out of your pantry. Children who feast on sugary foods wind up with little appetite for better food choices, so let sweets be a "once-in-a-while" snack. This way you'll help your child develop a taste for other foods.

If, like most kids, your child loves cereals, make sure to buy unsweetened varieties and sweeten them up with slices of fruit or raisins. At some point your child may beg you to buy some high-sugar, low-nutrition cereal. If you give in, "dilute" the sugary cereal with an equal amount of low-sugar, whole-grain cereal. Brush up on ways to sweeten foods without adding processed sugar. Fruit juices, unsweetened applesauce, and prune purees can be used in place of fats and sugars in many recipes.

While you're at it, ditch the caffeine as well. Caffeine doesn't belong in a child's diet. Since it's a stimulant, it can interfere with your child's concentration and ability to sleep well. Avoid soft drinks and iced tea, since these can contain large quantities of caffeine.

Remember to keep snack time healthful. Provide attractive, nutritious alternatives to high-calorie, low-nutrition packaged snack foods. A snack can be a little bit of a leftover meal or half a sandwich. Children love finger foods at snack time, so stock up on:

- bite-sized pieces of cheese or cheese sticks

- cut-up fresh veggies and fruit (beware of choke foods)
- dried fruits, such as raisins, figs, and prunes
- graham crackers and whole-grain crackers
- pretzels
- frozen fruit juice bars

Nutritional Supplements

If your child is eating a variety of healthful foods, he probably doesn't need dietary supplements of any kind.

Iron deficiency caused by nutritional inadequacy is unusual after age 2. However, if your child rarely eats meat, doesn't like iron-fortified cereals of any kind, and stays away from iron-rich vegetables, he may need additional iron and zinc. To boost your child's intake of iron without supplements, first try to get him to eat some of the following foods each week:

- liver
- beef
- dried beans
- dried fruit
- baked potatoes
- oatmeal
- iron-fortified cereals

Do not let your toddler or preschooler drink excessive amounts of milk (more than a quart per day). Too much milk can interfere with the absorption of iron and cause intestinal bleeding.

Some parents choose to give their child supplements. If you do, be sure to check labels for proper doses. If you have concerns or questions about vitamin or iron supplements, check with your doctor. He or she may also recommend a fluoride supplement for your child if you are using a nonfluoridated water supply. Be sure to store supplements well out of your child's reach; excessive amounts of supplements can poison a child.

Food Allergies

How will you know if your child is allergic to a newly introduced food or has developed an allergy to something he's been eating all along? The signs and symptoms of food allergies vary and can range from annoying to life threatening. Here are some symptoms that might indicate a food allergy:

- rashes, hives, and eczema
- respiratory ailments such as sneezing, coughing, a runny nose, and wheezing
- digestion problems, including vomiting, diarrhea, and abdominal pain
- Of course, these symptoms can be caused by problems other than a food allergy.

If your child has any of these symptoms, let your doctor know.

Most childhood food allergies can be traced back to five common foods: milk, eggs, peanuts, wheat, and soy. Shellfish, citrus fruits, and strawberries are also common causes of an allergic reaction. When the symptoms of food allergies are severe (such as difficulty breathing), your child will most likely need testing to pinpoint the exact problem. When the allergy is confined to a single food, such as peanuts, the offending food can simply be eliminated from a child's diet. If it turns out the child is allergic to all wheat products, or milk or eggs, you'll probably need a registered dietitian's help to plan a diet to meet your child's nutritional needs while avoiding those foods.

Healthy Mealtime Habits: 2 to 5 Years

For many children in this age group, food takes a backseat to the other wonders of a child's life - running, jumping, exploring. Just when it's time for children to begin eating adult foods in an adult manner, parents often have their hands full just trying to keep a toddler or preschooler sitting at the table!

What can you do to teach your child healthy eating habits and keep mealtimes pleasant and conflict-free? A good sense of humor can help, as can the suggestions below.

Healthy Mealtime Habits

At 2 years old, your child should be sharing conversation and good food with the rest of the family at mealtimes. Three well-balanced meals and two snacks a day should cover his nutritional requirements. The best news of all for Mom and Dad is that your toddler can feed himself. He's also quite adept at drinking from a cup, although you'll still want to opt for the type with a lid to cut back on spills. Your child's ability to feed himself will improve by age 3. By then, he'll be handling a fork well and might be trusted with a lidless cup. After age 3, you can direct your attention toward teaching table manners (don't talk with your mouth full, cut food into small bites, and so on), even though you've been showing your child by example all along.

Continue to be careful with foods your toddler can choke on, such as nuts, hot dogs, whole grapes, hard candies, large mouthfuls of peanut butter, and large pieces of raw vegetables. Chop or cut foods into small pieces, or wait until your child is better at chewing and swallowing. Since children this age are still prone to choke even on "safe" foods, don't leave your child alone while he is eating.

Family Meals

A child age 2 and older can join in the same healthy, well-balanced meals as the rest of the family, provided the child has not shown signs of any food allergies. Now might be a good time to recheck your own eating habits. Don't expect your child to want water with dinner if you're drinking soda. If you turn up your nose at fruits and vegetables, chances are your toddler will, too. For your child's sake, try expanding your food horizons at this time. You can help your toddler or preschooler develop his own good eating habits by:

buying a variety of healthy foods, including fruits, vegetables, and whole-grain breads and cereals allowing your child to choose from the variety of foods you provide

setting specific times for meals and snacks providing a healthy breakfast each morning

limiting sugary, high-fat snacks and drinks

(Not only do they contain little of nutritional value, they leave no room for healthy foods.)

avoiding adding excessive salt to foods encouraging your child to drink water, not just high-calorie fruit juices and empty-calorie sodas

avoiding caffeinated foods (such as chocolate) and drinks

sitting down and sharing mealtimes with your child

Wanting the same favorite foods at every meal is common at this age. As your child asserts his growing independence, he may even refuse these favorite foods occasionally, just to show you he can! Don't worry if your toddler or preschooler doesn't seem to have a balanced diet on a daily basis. As long as you keep offering a variety of healthful foods over the course of the week, your child should get the nutrition he needs. You can head off struggles at the table by offering new foods along with a food or two that you know your child likes. That way, you'll know your child will eat something, and the new foods will seem less scary. Provide small, easy-to-handle portions so your child won't be overwhelmed.

As your child grows, you can further encourage good eating habits by involving him in the grocery shopping, allowing him to help prepare and serve food, and getting him to set the table before meals. Continue to encourage your child to try a wide variety of new foods one at a time, but don't get discouraged if he sticks to old favorites. He'll surprise you one day by taking a bite! When introducing new foods, look for signs of allergic reaction. If you notice that your child develops a rash or has trouble breathing after eating any food, call your doctor right away.

Healthy Food Away From Home

Somewhere between ages 2 and 5, your child may start preschool and may begin visiting his friends' homes without you. Play dates with friends can be exciting and fun, especially if the friend's parents aren't as vigilant about sticking with healthy foods as Mom and Dad! Don't fret about the occasional soda or candy bar. Just make sure your child views them as "once-in-a-while" foods. Explain that some foods are better for him than others, and choosing nutritious foods is healthier.

If your child regularly eats snacks or meals at day care or preschool, find out what kinds of foods are served. Make sure the food is nutritious and the meals balanced. If you're not happy with the menus, contact the school or center director and express your concerns. Connect with other like-minded parents if you have trouble getting results yourself. Most parents want healthy foods for their kids and will press for a change if they become aware of problems.

Healthy Food Choices: 6 to 12 Years

As your child grows, continue to emphasize the main food groups, and strive to find choices from each group that your child enjoys. By the age of 5 or 6, a child can tell you pretty clearly what she likes and what she might be hungry for. Try to accommodate your child's tastes as much as possible, as long as the choices are within reason. Boys and girls between the ages of 6 and 10 require about 1,800 to 2,400 calories each day. This number rises considerably as children head into puberty. Girls begin to require about 200 calories per day more between the ages of 10 and 12. Boys start to need about 500 calories per day more after age 12. These additional calories and nutrients help fuel the incredible growth that occurs during adolescence.

Breads, cereals, rice, and pasta (6-11 servings)

Examples of servings:

1 slice of bread
½ bagel
¾ cup ready-to-eat cereal
½ cup cooked cereal
½ cup cooked pasta or rice
5-6 whole-grain crackers

Other good choices: cornbread, English muffins, reduced-fat muffins, low-salt, low-fat popcorn

Vegetables (3-5 servings)

Examples of servings:

¼ - ½ cup cooked vegetables
½ - 1 cup raw vegetables

Good choices: asparagus, beets, broccoli, carrots, cauliflower, corn, green and red peppers, green beans, lettuce and other greens, peas, potatoes, pumpkin, spinach, squash, sweet potatoes, tomatoes, vegetable juices, zucchini

Fruit (2-4 servings)

Examples of servings:

1 piece of fruit
½ cup canned fruit
½ cup juice

Good choices: apples, applesauce, apricots, bananas, cantaloupe, fruit cocktail, 100% fruit juices, grapefruit, kiwifruit, nectarines, oranges, peaches, plums, strawberries, watermelon

Dairy products (3 or 4 servings)

Examples of servings:

¾ - 1 cup low-fat or nonfat milk

1 - 1 ½ ounces low-fat or reduced-fat cheese

1 cup low-fat or nonfat yogurt

Other good choices: low-fat cottage cheese, ice milk, frozen yogurt, pudding

Meat, fish, poultry, and legumes (2 or 3 servings)

Examples of servings:

2 - 3 ounces of cooked lean meat, poultry, fish, or tofu

1 egg, ½ cup cooked dry beans, or 2 tablespoons of peanut butter counts as 1 ounce of lean meat

Other good choices: shellfish, dried peas, lentils, reduced-fat cold cuts

Facts on Fat and Fiber

Hopefully you've already reduced the fat in your child's diet. Although an adequate amount of dietary fat is crucial to development in very young children, dietary fat should begin to be reduced after age 2 or 3 to contribute only about 30% of the total calories for the day. Here are some ways to cut back:

Switch from whole milk to fat-free or nonfat (skim) milk or low-fat or light (1%) milk.

Serve more fish and poultry, and cut back on red meat.
Remove the skin from poultry, and trim fat from meats.
Reduce butter and margarine use.

Use low-fat cooking methods, such as baking, broiling, grilling, poaching, and steaming.

Serve fiber-rich foods, including whole-grain breads, cereals, dried peas and beans, fruits, and vegetables.

Fiber is an important nutritional component for children this age. Dietary fiber may play a role in reducing the chances of developing heart disease and cancer later in life. If you' provide the suggested servings of fruits and vegetables each day and serve whole-grain breads and cereals, you'll be well on the way toward ensuring your child gets enough dietary fiber.

The recommendation is to add 5 to your child's age to figure out how many grams of fiber she should be consuming each day. You can boost fiber intake by serving fresh salad with your meals, adding oat or wheat bran to any baked goods you make, and offering legumes such as chickpeas, lentils, and kidney beans at least once a week. Fiber intake should be increased gradually, though, since excessive fiber can cause painful bloating and gas. Don't forget to have your child drink plenty of water each day as well, since this can help reduce the chances of fiber-related intestinal discomfort. Be aware that excessive fiber intake can interfere with the body's absorption of crucial vitamins and minerals.

Calcium Counts

While calcium becomes even more important as puberty begins, it is important that school-age children get adequate amounts of dietary calcium to help ensure strong, healthy bones. Children ages 4 to 8 require 800 milligrams of calcium daily, while children ages 9 to 18 require 1,300 milligrams daily. You can meet these requirements by offering your children calcium-rich foods such as:

fat-free or nonfat (skim) milk or low-fat or light (1%) milk
low-fat or nonfat yogurt
low-fat or reduced-fat cheese
tofu
calcium-fortified fruit juices
ice cream and frozen yogurt (occasionally)

Taming the Sweet Tooth

Almost everyone has a sweet tooth, and that attraction to sweets makes it difficult to keep children from choosing candy, cookies, and cakes over healthier fare. You can't do much to take the sweet tooth out of the kid, but you can help control your child's access to sweets by keeping these foods out of your pantry. Children who feast on sugary foods wind up with little appetite for better food choices, so let sweets be a "once-in-a-while" snack. This way you'll help your child develop a taste for other foods. Brush up on ways to sweeten the taste of foods without adding processed sugar. Fruit juices, unsweetened applesauce, and prune purees can be used in place of fats and sugars in many recipes. While you're at it, ditch the caffeine as well. Caffeine doesn't belong in a child's diet. Since caffeine is a stimulant, it can interfere with your child's concentration and ability to sleep well. Avoid soft drinks and iced tea, since these beverages can contain large quantities of caffeine.

Nutritional Supplements

Many healthy children who eat a variety of good foods do not need supplements. Even the pickiest eater, given good food choices, will probably get what is needed over the course of a few days or a week. Check with your pediatrician if you're not sure that your child's diet provides the necessary nutrients.

Some parents choose to give their child supplements. In some cases, such as special dietary practices and certain medical conditions, a child's doctor may suggest a vitamin supplement. In either case, be sure to check labels for proper doses and appropriate amounts. If you have concerns or questions about the use of vitamin or mineral supplements, check with your doctor. He or she may also recommend a fluoride supplement for your child if you are using a nonfluoridated water supply. Be sure to store supplements well out of your child's reach; excessive amounts of some supplements can poison a child.

Healthy Mealtime Habits: 6-12 Years

Although the middle years of childhood are often seen as the calm between the tantrums of toddlerhood and the turmoil of adolescence, don't let up on your efforts when it comes to healthy eating. Continue to help your child understand the rewards of a strong and healthy body as she moves toward making an increasing number of decisions for herself. As your 6- to 12-year-old spends more of the day away from home and eats more meals and snacks away from your watchful eyes, providing her with the knowledge of how to make good food choices will become more important. At the same time, the meals you do share together will become a sort of "insurance policy" for your child, as these meals will provide the nutritious foods that can offset any empty-calorie fare consumed outside the home.

Family Meals

No doubt you've already discovered what an important role model you are to your child. In no area is this more apparent than nutrition. Today's busy families may not always have opportunities to share a meal together, but you should try to eat meals together as often as possible.

Getting together for meals provides many benefits. Here are a few:

- It enables you to act as a role model for good eating habits.
- It helps ensure that your child is eating nutritious foods.
- It allows you to find out your child's latest food likes and dislikes.
- It gives you an opportunity to introduce your child to new foods.
- It keeps you in tune with your child's triumphs and troubles.

The meals your child eats at home can set the tone for the meals she chooses on her own. You can continue to encourage good eating habits by:

- buying a variety of healthy foods, including fruits, vegetables, and whole-grain breads and cereals
- setting specific times for meals and snacks
- limiting sugary, high-fat snacks (Not only do they contain little of nutritional value, they leave no room for healthy foods.)

- avoiding adding excessive salt to foods
- encouraging your child to drink plenty of water, not just high-calorie fruit juices and empty-calorie sodas
- avoiding caffeine in the foods and drinks you serve your child
- setting a good example. You can't expect your child to choose water and an apple if you're snacking on colas and cookies.

Meals Away From Home

A child in this age group may be eating meals outside the home as often as (or more often than) she is eating at home. There may be snacks and lunch at school, birthday parties and sleepovers with friends, and scouting or sporting events that offer endless opportunities to eat. Will your child carry those good eating habits you've instilled out into the world? There are still a few things you can do to help:

- Make sure your child eats a nutritious breakfast.
- Send your child to school with a healthy lunch each day. Or, if food is provided at school, keep an eye on snack and lunch menus to make sure they meet your standards for nutrition. If they don't, make your concerns known to the appropriate staff at the school.
- Offer your child advice on how to choose healthy foods in a restaurant. Encourage her to include a salad or vegetables in her meals when ordering out.
- Continue to offer your child new and interesting foods at home, so that she has a wide variety of healthy choices when she is eating out.
- Allow your child to enjoy the birthday cake, ice cream, chocolate bars, and other treats that are such a sweet and memorable part of childhood. Simply make sure these foods are eaten in moderation, and balance the treats with more healthful fare at mealtimes.

Many children are fast-food fans, so remember to teach your child the benefits of choosing lower-fat selections. The typical cheeseburger, fries, and soda may be enticing, but encourage her to look for salads, grilled chicken sandwiches, and baked potatoes (without all the butter and sour cream). If your child simply must have that burger, suggest the simplest one on the menu rather than the double-decker, cheese-and-heavy-sauce-smothered advertised special. Fast-food restaurants offer milk and juice, too, so encourage your child to avoid the sodas and milk shakes. And remember to set a good example yourself. You'll be helping yourself as well as your youngster.

Another Healthy Habit: Exercise

Physical activity goes hand in hand with a good diet to help ensure a healthy body. Most children love to run and play and should be encouraged to do so each day. Encourage your child to replace television time with more physical activity. Don't count on your child's school day to provide enough activity - most do not. Also, don't count on group sports to give your child sufficient amounts of physical exertion. Practices and games rarely provide enough actual physical activity time per child to count toward a daily exercise routine. Rather, plan activities for the whole family that get you up and moving. Try:

- dancing together to the radio
- playing on the backyard swingset or at the local playground
- swimming
- taking a family run or walk
- riding bikes (Don't forget to wear helmets!)
- in-line skating or ice skating (Don't forget to wear helmets!)
- playing tag
- running relay races
- flying a kite
- playing catch

Set a good example by taking part in an exercise program yourself, whether alone or with your kids. Whatever activity you do together, remember to make exercise fun so it becomes an important and pleasant part of your child's life.

Breakfast

Whether your child chows down on a full breakfast at home, eats a brown-bag breakfast on the ride to school, or buys a cafeteria breakfast once she gets there, there is no meal that is more important than the first one of the day. Studies show that kids who skip breakfast or eat unhealthy foods, like doughnuts or pastries, can have a hard time concentrating just a few hours later. To head off this problem, find foods your child likes to eat and serve them in the morning, even if they're not "traditional" breakfast fare. Let your child giggle over spaghetti, a peanut butter and jelly sandwich, or leftover pizza at 7 a.m. These options beat sugary cereals and cakes nutritionally, and they will help your child do her best all morning long, whether at school or play.

If, like most kids, your child loves cereals, buy the lower-sugar or unsweetened varieties and sweeten them up with slices of fruit or raisins. At some point your child may ask you to buy some high-sugar, low-nutrition cereal. If you give in, "dilute" the sugary cereal with an equal amount of a nutritious whole-grain cereal.

"What's for lunch, Mom?"

If you pack lunches for your child each day, you already know it can be a challenge to send foods that are healthy and appealing. One idea to overcome this challenge is to involve your youngster in the preparation. Ask your child to help pack her lunch box, encouraging her to pack healthy foods she enjoys as well as the occasional treat. This activity of selecting her own lunch may make your child less likely to trade her food for less nutritious items her friends may have or to throw it away.

Teach your child that a bag lunch needs to be well-rounded by packing something from each of the food groups: protein, grains, fruits, vegetables, and dairy. Here are some healthful ideas:

- For protein, try water-packed tuna, sliced ham or turkey, bean chili, baked beans, peanut butter, or hard-boiled eggs.
- For grains, try whole-wheat breads and crackers, low-fat bran muffins, or pretzels.
- For fruits and vegetables, try sliced fresh fruit, carrot and celery sticks, or a thermos of cooked vegetables.
- For dairy, try a thermos of low-fat milk, a container of low-fat yogurt, low-fat cheese, or a scoop of low-fat cottage cheese.

Snacks

Kids in this age group are often "super-snackers." If this is the case with your school-age child, you'll want to emphasize healthy food choices at snack time, since a lot of unwanted fat and calories can creep into a child's diet through snacks. The best idea, especially for today's hectic households, is to keep good-tasting, good-for-you foods close and accessible. Ask your child what she'd like to have on hand. Maximize the nutritional value of snack time by combining a few of the ideas below:

- microwave popcorn (low-salt, low-fat variety)
- fresh fruit
- celery and carrot sticks with low-fat dip or dressing
- raisins and other dried fruits
- low-fat or nonfat miik and yogurt
- low-sugar cereals
- unsweetened applesauce
- frozen fruit juice on a stick
- frozen bananas
- graham crackers
- fresh fruit juice
- pretzels
- "trail mix" - dried fruit, nuts, low-sugar cereal, mini-pretzels

Dinner

You can keep dinner interesting by allowing your child to participate in the planning and purchasing of meals. Encourage your child to design menus, choosing at least one favorite food for each meal, and then take her to the supermarket to buy food for the week. As you shop, explain the choices you make. Teach your child that many of the most attractively packaged and promoted foods are often empty-calorie and highly processed fare. You and your child can read food labels together and learn how to compare the nutritional content of different foods and different brands. Once again, you are giving your child the tools to make healthy food choices for the rest of her life.

Your child can start to help out in the kitchen, too: teach her how to wash and trim vegetables and measure and pour ingredients. Instruct your child on food safety and the safe use of the microwave and stove. By age 10, many kids are comfortable cooking and can be trusted with small heating or baking chores, as long as an adult is close by. Simply being involved in the preparation can make a meal tastier to a child.

Don't cater to a finicky eater by cooking special meals just for her. Make sure your child doesn't go hungry even if she snubs the main dish by including something in the meal that you know she likes. A slice of bread, piece of fruit, or a helping of potatoes will tide her over to the next meal or snack. Let her know that it is not acceptable if she complains about individual dishes she dislikes. Make it clear that she may not ruin the meal for the rest of the family and that she will not be eating anything else until the next scheduled snack or meal.

Special Nutritional Concerns: Children Age 6 to 12

Overweight Children

About 25% to 30% of American school-age children are overweight, which puts them at risk for disease and low self-esteem. Is your child at risk? One way to know for sure is to check with your pediatrician, who will determine if your child is more than 20% above the ideal weight for her height and age. If your child is moderately overweight, there will probably be no talk of dieting at this age. Instead, the emphasis will be on lowering the rate of weight gain as the child grows taller. Stalling weight gain can be accomplished by changing eating habits, lowering fat intake, and increasing a child's level of physical activity. Don't punish or scold your child - use positive reinforcement. Make physical activity fun and rewarding, and involve the entire family.

If a child is more than 40% overweight, a doctor-guided weight loss program may be suggested. During the course of the program, the emphasis should be on adopting a healthier lifestyle for the long term, not just on losing weight now. No matter what your children's size or shape, help them love themselves by praising their positive strengths and skills. It is important to de-emphasize weight and emphasize feeling healthy and strong. Above all, never put a child in this age group on a diet without consulting your doctor first. Restricting a child's diet too much can interfere with growth and development. A registered dietitian who specializes in pediatrics can be a big help.

Eating Disorders

Eating disorders are of special concern as children head into adolescence at the end of this period. Young girls seem to be particularly at risk for developing a poor body image. They see society's obsession with thinness and then starve themselves (anorexia nervosa) or binge and purge (bulimia). Although eating disorders are generally not a problem until after puberty begins, parents should be alert to any danger signs an older school-age child exhibits. Preoccupation with weight and size, a drastic reduction in food intake, or a lack of weight gain despite a large appetite can mean a child may have an eating disorder. Check with your pediatrician for help, since eating disorders can lead to serious health problems and even death. Counseling can successfully guide these children through this risky time.

Young Athletes

While all parents of school-age kids should be stressing the importance of physical activity, it's also important to monitor the eating habits of young athletes. Although everything possible should be done to offer them optimal nutrition to support their efforts, it's also crucial to avoid some risky behavior often associated with the search for a competitive edge. Your child's athletic performance depends on the same balanced diet that will keep her noncompetitive classmates sharp. Make sure your budding baseball star or soccer lover is getting enough calories to support her level of physical exertion. You can do this by adding carbohydrates, such as potatoes, rice, pasta, and beans, to your child's diet. These are excellent sources of energy.

Teaching your child, especially your athlete, to enjoy water is one of the healthiest gifts you can give. Children should be urged to drink plenty of water before exercise and every 10 minutes or so during their activity. For every half hour of strenuous activity, your child should drink an extra 8 to 12 ounces of water - the drink of choice. When drinking sports drinks, avoid those that are high in sugar, which can cause cramping, nausea, and diarrhea. Also, make sure your child balances practice and performance with adequate rest and relaxation. These are as necessary to well-being as proper nutrition.

Does Your Child Need Vitamin Supplements?

Vitamins and minerals are important elements of the total nutritional requirements of your child. Because the human body itself is unable to produce adequate amounts of many vitamins, they must be obtained from the diet. The body needs these vitamins in only tiny amounts, and in a balanced diet they are usually present in sufficient quantities in the foods your youngster eats. Thus, in middle childhood, supplements are rarely needed.

For some youngsters, however, pediatricians may recommend a daily supplement. If your child has a poor appetite or erratic eating habits, or if she consumes a highly selective diet (such as a vegetarian diet containing no dairy products), a vitamin supplement should be considered. Chewable tablets are available for children who have difficulty swallowing pills.

These over-the-counter supplements are generally safe; nonetheless, they are drugs. If taken in excessive amounts (in tablets, capsules or combined with other supplements), some supplements - particularly the fat-soluble vitamins (A, D, E and K) - can be toxic. Scientists are finding that in some special situations and diseases, vitamin supplementation can be an important contributor to health. However, so-called megavitamin therapy or orthomolecular medicine - in which vitamins are given in extremely large doses for conditions ranging from mental retardation to hyperactivity to dyslexia - has no proven scientific validity and may pose some risks. Vitamin C, for example, when consumed in megadoses in hopes of undermining a cold, can sometimes cause headaches, diarrhea, nausea and cramps. Always consult your pediatrician before giving your child supplements. And don't leave a bottle of vitamins on the table as though they were a condiment like salt or pepper; taking vitamins should be done with careful consideration.

Sources for Various Vitamins and Minerals

As much as possible, try to maximize the vitamins your child receives in her regular meals. Following are some of the vitamins and minerals necessary for normally growing children, and some of the foods that contain them.

Vitamin A promotes normal growth, healthy skin, and tissue repair, and aids in night and color vision. Rich sources include yellow vegetables, dairy products and liver.

The B vitamins promote red blood cell formation and assist in a variety of metabolic activities. They are found in meat (including liver), poultry, fish, soybeans, milk, eggs, whole grains and enriched breads and cereals.

Vitamin C strengthens connective tissue, muscles, and skin, hastens the healing of wounds and bones and increases resistance to infection. Vitamin C is found in citrus fruits, strawberries, tomatoes, potatoes, Brussels sprouts, spinach and broccoli.

Vitamin D promotes tooth and bone formation and regulates the absorption of minerals like calcium. Sources include fortified dairy products, fish oils, fortified margarine and egg yolks. Although vitamin proponents insist that large doses of vitamin D - far greater than the U.S. Recommended Daily Allowances - can build even stronger bones, there is no evidence to support this claim, and excessive quantities of vitamin D are potentially toxic. Sunlight also contributes to dietary sources of vitamin D, stimulating the conversion of a naturally occurring compound in the skin to an active form of the vitamin.

Especially during periods of rapid growth, iron is essential for the production of blood and the building of muscles. When iron levels are low, your child may demonstrate symptoms such as irritability, listlessness, depression and an increased susceptibility to infection. However, a deficiency of iron is much more common in adolescence than in middle childhood. Once girls begin menstruation, they need much more iron than boys do. The best sources of iron include beef, turkey, pork and liver. Spinach, beans and prunes also contain modest amounts of iron. Some cereals and flour are enriched with iron.

As your child matures, calcium is necessary for healthy bone development. An inadequate calcium intake during childhood can not only affect present growth but might also help contribute to the development of weakened and porous bones (osteoporosis) later in life. Low-fat milk, cheese, yogurt and sardines are excellent sources of calcium. Some vegetables, such as broccoli and spinach, also contain modest amounts of calcium. Some fruit juices are now fortified and provide a good source of calcium

Failure to Thrive

For purchasing or reprint information, click here.

If you plot your child's weight and measurements, you should see a continuous upward trend, although there will be times when she gains very slowly and perhaps some weeks when she actually loses a little weight due to illness. It is not normal for her to stop growing, or to decrease in weight except for the small amount she loses during the first few days of life. If she does lose weight, it's a clear sign either that she's not getting enough to eat or that she's ill. The medical term for this condition is failure to thrive. Although it can occur in older children who are seriously ill or undernourished, it is most common and most dangerous during the active growth period of the first three years.

If allowed to continue for a prolonged period, this condition can become serious. Steady weight gain is especially important for infants and toddlers because it indicates that they are receiving adequate nutrition and care for normal physical, mental and emotional development.

Causes of Failure to Thrive

Usually when a child stops growing, it's due to a feeding problem that prevents her from getting as many calories as she needs. As a newborn, she may be too fussy to eat as much as she needs, or, if breastfed, she may not be getting enough milk while nursing. Some children may require more food than their parents are able to provide. These problems must be detected and treated early in order to avoid long-term or permanent damage.

Sometimes failure to thrive signals a medical problem. The newborn may have an infection passed on from her mother during pregnancy, or she may have a hormonal difficulty, allergy or a digestive problem that prevents nutrients from being properly absorbed into the body. Diseases such as diabetes, cystic fibrosis or heart disease also can interfere with normal growth. If one of these is present, the child may need a special diet as well as medical treatment.

When to Call the Pediatrician for Failure to Thrive

Regular charting of your child's growth and comparison of her general development with others her age is the best way to make sure she is thriving. If she does not gain weight, grow in length, or otherwise develop normally, consult your pediatrician, who will measure and examine your child, ask about her diet and eating patterns, and review her medical history for signs of illness that may be contributing to her failure to thrive. The physician will try to establish exactly when the growth or weight gain stopped, and ask about any incidents or events that may have contributed to this. The pediatrician may watch the youngster eating or nursing to see how much she consumes and how she responds to food. Sometimes a short period of in-hospital observation may be necessary.

If the doctor discovers a physical cause for the decrease in growth rate, the appropriate treatment will be

recommended. If there is no physical reason; however, the pediatrician will look for emotional or social problems, particularly within the family. Such disturbances can decrease a child's appetite or alter her normal food intake and digestion. Once discovered, these difficulties can be treated with individual or family counseling.

CHAPTER 8

HEALTHY INDIAN RECIPES

Baked Vegetable Jalfrazie

Preparation time: 15 minutes * Cooking time: 30 minutes * Serves 8.

Ingredients

1 teacups chopped mixed boiled vegetables (French beans, carrots, cauliflower, green peas)

2 chopped onions
4 tablespoons chopped capsicum
1 chopped tomatoes
½ to 1 teaspoon chili powder a pinch garam masala
2 tablespoons chopped coriander
4 tablespoons grated paneer, plus a little extra for topping
1-1/2 teacup tomato gravy
4 teaspoons oil - Salt to taste

Heat the oil and fry the onions for ½ minute. Add the capsicum and tomatoes and fry again for 2 minutes. Add the vegetables, chilli powder, garam masala, coriander and salt and cook for a few minutes. pread the tomato gravy on top and sprinkle a little grated paneer over it. Bake in a hot oven at 200C for 10 minutes * Serve hot.

Health Information: This recipe uses baking, a superior technique of cooking, instead of sautéing or frying in oil.

Per Serving: Calories 86 * Protein 4g * Carbohydrates 9g * Fat 3.8g

Besan ka Cheela

Preparation Time: 15 minutes * Cooking Time: 2 minutes

Ingredients
2 cups Besan
1 large Onion finely chopped
1 Green Chilli finely chopped
1 bunch Coriander leaves finely chopped
1tsp.Ajwain.

1 tsp. Black Pepper powder
½ tsp. Red Chilli powder
1 tsp. Chat Masala
1 tsp. Coriander powder
Salt to taste

1- 1 ½ cup water approximately to make a smooth batter.
Oil for cooking.

Put all the ingredients except water in a big bowl. Now start adding small quantities of water to make a smooth batter, so that there should be no lumps in it. Add water till it comes to a dropping consistency or just like dosa batter. Now keep it aside.

Now heat a non-stick- tawa or heavy bottom frying pan, then turn the heat on medium. Put little oil on tawa [1tsp.] & spread 1 serving spoonful of batter evenly on it. Cover it with lid just for a minute so that it should cook inside also. Then remove lid, put some more oil on the top & turn it upside down. Let it be brown & crispy from both sides.

Repeat the same with rest of the batter. Serve hot with Green Chutney or Sause. It can be taken with toast also.

- Serve hot and eat as you wish and Enjoy

Per Cheela: Calories: 80 per cheela

Bhurta Salad

Preparation time: 5 minutes * Cooking time: 15 minutes * Serves 4.

Ingredients

½ kg. large round brinjals
1 chopped onion
1 teaspoon finely chopped green chilli
1 chopped tomato
2 teaspoons oil
Salt to taste

Grill the brinjals on a fire until they become black in colour. Remove the skin and mesh thoroughly. Heat the oil and fry the onion for ½ minute. Add the green chilli and fry again for a few seconds. Add the tomato and fry again for 2 minutes. Add the meshed brinjals and salt. Add ½ teacup beaten fresh curds, and a pinch of sugar to the above mixture. * Serve cold

Health Information: A light dish for the brinjal lovers. Rich in vitamins and minerals.

Per Serving: Calories 69 * Protein 2g * Carbohydrates 10g * Fat 2.8g

Brinjal Bhurta

Preparation time: 5 minutes * Cooking time: 15 minutes * Serves 4.

Ingredients

½ kg. large round brinjals

1 chopped onion
1 teaspoon finely chopped green chilli
1 chopped tomato
2 teaspoons oil
Salt to taste

Grill the brinjals on a fire until they become black in colour. Remove the skin and mesh thoroughly.

Heat the oil and fry the onion for ½ minute.

Add the green chilli and fry again for a few seconds.

Add the tomato and fry again for 2 minutes.

Add the meshed brinjals and salt.

- Serve hot.

Variation: BHURTA SALAD Add ½ teacup beaten fresh curds, and a pinch of sugar to the above mixture. Serve cold as a salad.

Health Information: A light dish for the brinjal lover. Rich in vitamins and minerals.

Per Serving: Calories 69 * Protein 2g * Carbohydrates 10g * Fat 2.8g

Cabbage Stuffing for Plain Parathas

Preparation Time: 10 minutes, * No Cooking, * For 12 Parathas

Ingredients
3 teacups finely chopped cabbage
2 teaspoons crumbled paneer
1 chopped green chilli
2 tablespoons chopped coriander
Salt to taste

Sprinkle 1 teaspoon of salt over the cabbage. Leave for 10 minutes and then squeeze out the water. Add the remaining ingredients and mix well.

Health Information: Besides being one of the best sources of Vitamin C, cabbage also provides calcium, phosphorous and potassium. It is good for growing children.

Per Paratha: Calories: 10, * Protein: 1 g * Carbohydrates: 2g * Fat: 0g

Cauliflower Stuffing for Plain Parathas

Preparation Time: 10 minutes, * Cooking Time: A few minutes * For 12 Parathas

Ingredients
2 teacups grated cauliflower
½ teaspoon cumin seeds
1 chopped onion
2 chopped green chilis
1 teaspoon chilli powder (optional)
1 tablespoons chopped coriander
2 teaspoons oil
Salt to taste
Heat the oil and fry the cumin seeds for ½ minute
Add the onion, green chilies and fry again for ½ minute

Add the cauliflower and salt, sprinkle a little water and cook until three-quarters cooked

Add the chili powder and coriander and mix well

Health Information: A tasty filling which will increase the Vitamin C and fibre content of parathas.

Per Paratha: Calories: 15 * Protein: 0.5g * Carbohydrates: 1.5g * Fat: 0.9g

Chinese Stuffing for Plain Parathas

Preparation Time: 10 minutes, * Cooking Time: 5 minutes, * For 10 Parathas

Ingredients
1 teacup coarsely grated carrots
1-1/2 teacups shredded cabbage
4 teaspoons bean sprouts (optional)
1 sliced onion
a pinch baking powder
a few drops soya sauce
a pinch of sugar
1 tablespoon oil
Salt to taste

Heat the oil on a high flame

Add the carrots, cabbage, bean sprouts, onion and baking powder and cook on a high flame for 3 to 4 minutes.

Add the soya sauce, sugar and salt..

Health Information: A paratha stuffing with an Oriental flavour using the nutrient saving stir-frying method of cooking.

Per Paratha: Calories: 39 * Protein: 1g * Carbohydrates: 5g * Fat: 1.6g

Dal with Spinach

Preparation time: 10 minutes * Cooking time: 25 minutes * Serves 8.

Ingredients

¾ teacup uncooked moong dal or masoor dal

1 chopped onion

1 teaspoon cumin seeds

1 teacup chopped spinach

2 teaspoons amchur powder

1 chopped tomato

½ teaspoon turmeric powder

4 teaspoons oil

Salt to taste

To be ground into a paste

6 cloves garlic

3 green chilies

25 mm. piece of ginger

Cook the dal in 3 teacups of water.

Heat the oil, add the onion and cumin seeds and fry for 2 minutes.

Add the cooked dal, the spinach, amchur powder, tomato, turmeric powder, paste and salt and boil for 5 minutes.

- Serve hot.

Health Information: This recipe of dal enriched with spinach is a very good source of pretein. The garlic used for flavouring is known for its medicinal properties and acts as an antibacterial agent.

Per Serving: Calories 90 * Protein 5g * Carbohydrates 12g * Fat 2.9g

Masoor Dal with Rice

Preparation Time: 10 minutes, * Cooking Time: 40 minutes, * Serves 4

Ingredients

100 grams uncooked rice

½ teacup uncooked masoor or tur dal

1 teaspoons cumin seeds

2 slit green chilies
100 grams cauliflower pieces
2 tablespoons diced carrots
¼ teaspoon turmeric powder
1 sliced tomato
1 tablespoon chopped coriander
2 teaspoons ghee
Salt to taste
Cook the rice. Cool and keep aside
Cook the dal in a pressure cooker. Add 2-1/2 teacups of water to the cooked dal and beat well

Heat the ghee and fry the cumin seeds for a while

Add the onion slices and green chilies and cook for a while

Add the cooked dal, cauliflower, carrots, turmeric and salt and cook for 10 minutes on a slow flame

Finally, add the tomato and chopped coriander and cook for a few minutes

- Serve the dal with the cooked rice.

Health Information: The protein contained in rice and dal complement each other to give a higher quality protein which is the corner stone of our nutritious meal. Be sure not to rinse the rice more than required to remove the dirt since excess washing will result in loss of vitamins.

Per Serving: Calories: 188 * Protein: 7g * Carbohydrates: 34g * Fat: 3.5g

Minty Stuffed Parathas

Preparation Time: 30 minutes * Cooking Time: 45 minutes * Makes 20 parathas

Ingredients
For the dough
2 teacups whole wheat flour
½ teaspoon salt
2 teaspoon oil
For the mint sauce (for the dough)

¾ teacup mint leaves
1 teaspoon lemon juice

½ level teaspoon cumin seeds
3 green chilies
1 level teaspoon salt
For the Stuffing

2 teacups chopped cabbage
1 teacup boiled green peas
1 chopped potato
1 chopped onion
Juice of 1 lemon
2 pinches garam masala
1 tablespoon chopped coriander
1 tablespoon ground green chili
½ level teaspoon sugar
2 teaspoons oil
Salt to taste
For Cooking

2 teaspoons oil or butter
Accompaniment

1-1/2 teacups fresh curds (optional)
For the dough
Pour all the ingredients for the sauce with ½ teacup of water into a mixer and blend

Mix the mint sauce with the wheat flour, oil and salt and prepare a soft dough

Knead well and divide into 20 portions. Roll out the portions into thin rotis

For the Stuffing

Sprinkle salt over the cabbage and leave aside for 10 minutes. Thereafter, squeeze out the water from the cabbage using your hands

Crush the green peas

Heat the oil and add the potato and crushed peas. Sprinkle a little water on top, cover and cook until soft

Add the cabbage and onion and cook for 1 minute

Add the lemon juice, garam masala, coriander, green chili, sugar and salt.

Divide into 20 portions
How to proceed

Put one portion of the stuffing on each roti and fold.

Arrange all the stuffed rotis in a greased baking tray

Brush lightly with a little ghee or butter and bake in a hot oven at 200 degree Celsius until pink spots appear

Health Information: A high fibre paratha having complex carbohydrates which are a better kind of energy supply than the simple carbohydrates obtained from pure sugar. An excellent recipe for athletes who need complex carbohydrates and a little fat.

Per Paratha: Calories: 91 * Protein: 3g * Carbohydrates: 17g * Fat: 1.4g

Mixed Pulses with Vegetables

Preparation Time: 20 minutes * Cooking Time: 50 minutes * Serves 8

Ingredients

2 tablespoons whole moong
2 tablespoons gram (chana)
1 tablespoons whole masoor
175 grams cauliflower
6 to 7 small whole onions
2 sliced onions
2 large chopped tomatoes
3 teaspoons ghee
Salt to taste
1 sliced tomato and 1 tablespoon chopped coriander for decoration

To be ground into a paste

8 cloves garlic
8 red chilies
2 teaspoons coriander seeds
2 teaspoons cumin seeds
25 mm piece ginger
Soak the moong, gram and masoor in water for at least 6 hours. Drain and allow to sprout for 12 hours

Add 2 teacups of water and cook in a pressure cooker

Cut the cauliflower into big pieces and boil with whole onions

How to Proceed

Heat the oil and fry the sliced onions for 3 minutes
Add the paste and fry again for 3 to 4 minutes
Add the soaked pulses and cook for a few minutes
Add the cauliflower, whole onions, tomatoes and salt and cook for at least 10 minutes. If you like, add 3 to 4 teaspoons of tamarind water before serving.

- Serve hot decorated with tomato slices and chopped coriander.

Health Information: This combination of pulses and mixed vegetables gives a protein rich dish

Per Serving: Calories: 88 * Protein: 4g * Carbohydrates: 13g * Fat: 2.6g

Moong Dal Dahi Vadas

Preparation Time: 15 minutes * Cooking Time: 15 minutes * Makes 8 Vadas

Ingredients

½ teacup moong dal (with skin)
2 green chilies
A pinch of Asafoetida
½ teaspoon soda bi-carb or fruit salt
2 teacups fresh curds
2 pinches roasted cumin powder
2 pinches chili powder
1 tablespoon chopped coriander (optional)
Salt to taste
For the Seasoning

½ teaspoon mustard seeds
3 to 4 pieces green chilies
A pinch of Asafoetida
1-1/2 teaspoons oil
Soak the moong dal for 3 to 4 hours. Drain

Add the green chilies and blend in a mixer with very little water

Add the asafoetida and soda bi-carb and mix well

Heat a non-stick sandwich toaster and spread 1 teaspoon of the mixture in each cavity. Close the heat. When ready, the mixture will be toasted into pieces of triangular shape. Take out the toasts

Dip the toasts in water for 5 minutes. Thereafter, squeeze out the water and arrange the vadas on a plate

Beat the curds with the salt

To prepare the seasoning, heat the oil and fry the mustard seeds for ½ minute. Add the green chilies and asafoetida. Mix the seasoning with the beaten curds

- Spread the seasoned curds over the vadas. Sprinkle the cumin powder, chili powder and coriander on top and serve. If you like, also sprinkle sweet and sour chutney

Health Information: Instead of the traditional method of frying dahi vadas, this recipe uses a different cooking technique to give a healthier dish which is lower in calories and fat.

Per Vada: Calories: 61 * Protein: 4.5g * Carbohydrates: 7.5g * Fat: 1.6g

Moong Dal Dhoklas

Preparation Time: 20 minutes * Cooking Time: 20 minutes * Makes 16 pieces

Ingredients How to ?
1 teacup moong dal with skin
2 teaspoon gram flour (besan)
2 green chilies
1tablespoon fresh curds
2 teaspoons fruit salt
A pinch asafoetida
Salt to taste
For the topping

2 tablespoons finely chopped cabbage
2 tablespoons finely chopped carrots
Soak the moong dal for 2 hours. Drain
Add the green chilies and a little water and grind in a mixer
Add the gram flour, curds, asafoetida and salt
When you want to serve, add the fruit salt and mix well
Pour the mixture into 2 thalis of about 200 mm diameter.
Sprinkle the cabbage on top and steam for 5 minutes

- Serve Hot

Health Information: A protein rich Gujarati speciality without oil. Excellent with meals of for breakfast or tea-time.

Per Paratha: Calories: 36 * Protein: 3g * Carbohydrates: 6g * Fat: 0.4g

Moong Dal Panki

Preparation Time: 10 minutes * Cooking Time: 10 minutes * Makes 8 pankies

Ingredients

50 grams moong dal
1 tablespoon fresh curds
2 green chilies
1 teaspoon gram flour (besan)
A pinch Asafoetida
1 tablespoon chopped coriander
A pinch sugar
½ teaspoon lemon juice
Salt to taste
Soak the moong dal in water for 2 hours. Drain.
Grind with the fresh curds and green chilies
Add the gram flour, asafoetida
Grease balana leaves lightly
Spread 1 tablespoon of the mixture on one leaf and cover with another leaf. Roast on a tawa (griddle) until brown spots appear on both sides.

- Serve hot with green chutney

Health Information: An excellent low calorie snack which is a good source of protein.

Per Panki: Calories: 28 * Protein: 2g * Carbohydrates: 5g * Fat: 0.3g

Moong Misal

Preparation Time: 10 minutes * Cooking Time: 5 minutes * Serves 6

Ingredients
1 teacup sprouted moong
1 teacup fresh curds
4 teaspoons sweet and sour chutney
2 chopped tomatoes
2 chopped onions
A little cumin seed powder
2 teaspoons oil
Salt and chili powder to taste
Heat the oil, add the moong, ½ teacup of water and salt. Cover and cook on a low flame until the moong is soft

Beat the curds with a pinch of salt
How to Serve
Spread the hot moong on a serving plate. Top with the beaten curds, the chutney, tomatoes, onions, cumin seed powder, chili powder and salt

Serve immediately

Health Information: The recipe combines the proteins of moong beans and a dairy product so as to make the proteins complete

Per Serving: Calories: 87 * Protein: 5g * Carbohydrates: 12.5g * Fat: 2.5g

Nawabi Curry

Preparation time: 25 minutes * Cooking time: 15 minutes * Serves 6.

Ingredients
3 large tomatoes
100 grams finely chopped mixed boiled vegetables. (French beans, carrots, cauliflower)

½ teaspoon sugar

1 tablespoon oil Salt to taste To be ground into a paste

1 large onion

1 tablespoon coriander seeds

1 tablespoon cumin seeds

1 tablespoon khus-khus

2 teaspoons aniseed

25 mm piece of ginger

2 green chilies

3 cardamoms

3 cloves

2 sticks cinnamon

Accompaniment: Plain parathas

Chop the tomatoes. Add 1-1/2 teacups of water and cook until soft

Pass through a sieve to make a tomato puree.

Heat the oil and fry the paste for 2 to 3 minutes.

Add the tomato puree, vegetables, sugar and salt.

Serve hot with plain parathas

Note: Each plain paratha contains 54 calories.

Health Information: A royal curry that is low in calories and goes wonderfully with parathas. A combination of herbs and spices brings out the taste with less salt.

Per Serving: Calories 66 * Protein 2g * Carbohydrates 7g * Fat 3.9g

Paneer Methi Palak

Preparation time: 10 minutes * Cooking time: 20 minutes * Serves 5.

Ingredients

1 teacups chopped spinach

1 teacup fresh fenugreek (methi) leaves a pinch soda bi-carb

25 mm. piece of ginger

1 chopped onion

3 chopped green chilies
100 grams sliced paneer
3 teaspoons oil
Salt to taste

Chop the spinach and fenugreek leaves finely.

Add 2 teaspoons of water and the soda bi-carb and cook on a slow flame until soft.

When cooked, drain out the water and blend the leaves in a liquidizer.

Chop the ginger finely.

Heat the oil and fry the onion for 1 minute.

Add the green chilies and ginger and fry again for a few seconds.

Add the blended leaves, paneer and salt.

- Serve hot

Health Information: Green leafy vegetables contain Vitamins A and C and iron and form an important part of a balanced diet. The paneer provides high quality protein.

Per Serving: Calories 88 * Protein 9g * Carbohydrates 6.5g * Fat 3.6g

Paneer Palak Methi Rotis

Preparation Time: 10 minutes * Cooking Time: 15 minutes * Makes 6 rotis

Ingredients
For the dough
1 teacup whole wheat flour
1 teaspoon oil
½ teacup finely chopped fenugreek (methi) leaves and palak
1 tablespoon fresh curds
½ teaspoon chili powder
¼ teaspoon turmeric powder
A pinch asafoetida
½ teaspoon sugar
Salt to taste
For the topping

½ teacup finely chopped fenugreek (methi) leaves and palak

1 tablespoon grated paneer

For the dough

Mix the ingredients and knead into a dough. Add more curds if required to make the dough

Divide into 6 portions and roll out into rotis
Cook on a tawa (griddle) on both sides
How to proceed
When you want to serve, sprinkle a little topping on top of each roti. Place below the grill for 1 minute.

- Serve Hot

Health Information: Methi, palak and paneer, when added to the whole wheat chapatti increase the calcium content more than 7 times. Methi is rich in calcium and Vitamins A and C

Per Paratha: Calories: 90 * Protein: 4g * Carbohydrates: 16g * Fat: 1.4g

Plain Parathas

Preparation time: 10 minutes * Cooking time: a few minutes * Makes 12 thin parathas

Ingredients

For the dough
1 teacup whole wheat flour
¼ teaspoon salt
1 teaspoon oil

For cooking

2 teaspoons melted butter

Accompaniment
1 teacup fresh curd
For making dough

Mix all the ingredients and enough water to make a soft dough.

Divide the dough into 12 portions and roll out each portion into very thin 150mm diameter rounds.

Cook on a tawa (griddle) very lightly for a few seconds.

Put a portion of the desired stuffing in each paratha and fold. Arrange on a greased baking tray.

Brush the parathas lightly with butter and bake in a hot oven at 200 deg C until light pink in colour (about 5 minutes). Alternatively, cook on a tawa (griddle) on both sides and brush lightly with butter or oil.

Serve hot with curd.

Note: 1 teacup fresh curd contains 63 calories i.e.5 calories per serving.

Health Information: Whole grain flour contains more vitamins, minerals and fibre as compared to highly refined flour where most of the vitamins and minerals are destroyed during processing. When parathas or chapattis are combined with a small amount of pulses and beans or with a dairy product like curds, the amino acids in these complement each other to give a higher quality of protein

Per Paratha: Calories 54 *Protein: 2g * Carbohydrates: g * Fat: 1.5 g

Pumpkin Handva

Preparation Time: 10 minutes * Cooking Time: 15 minutes * Serves 5

Ingredients

3 teacups grated white pumpkin (lauki)
5 tablespoons coarse jowar flour
1 chopped green chili
2 tablespoons chopped coriander
¼ teaspoons soda bi-carb
2 pinches sugar
Salt to taste
For the topping

1 chopped tomato
1 chopped onion

2 tablespoons tomato ketchup or sweet and sour sauce

Squeeze out a little water from the pumpkin. Add the flour, green chili, coriander, soda bi-carb, sugar and salt and mix well

Spread the mixture on a baking tray and bake in a hot oven at 225 degree Celsius for 15 minutes. Top with the tomato, onion and ketchup or sweet and sour sauce

- Cut into pieces and Serve

Health Information: Pumpkin contains 96% water and makes this traditional Gujarati dish low in calories. Jowar contains more iron than wheat flour. It also imparts an unusual flavour to the handva

Per Serving: Calories: 79 * Protein: 2g * Carbohydrates: 17g * Fat: 03.5g

Rice and Moong Dal Idli

Preparation Time: 20 minutes * Cooking Time: 30 minutes * Serves 8

Ingredients

½ teacup rice
½ teacup moong dal
¼ teaspoon fenugreek (methi) seeds (optional)
A pinch soda bi-carb
Salt to taste

Soak the rice, dal and fenugreek seeds in water for 5 to 6 hours

Grind the soaked ingredients in a mixer and leave the batter aside for at least 8 hours or preferably overnight

Thereafter, add the soda bi-carb and salt and pour a little mixture into the cavities of a small idli maker

Steam in a cooker for a few minutes. Repeat for the remaining mixture

Serve hot with chutney

Health Information: This novel combination gives idlis having a different flavour and a high protein content.

Per Serving: Calories: 66 * Protein: 3g * Carbohydrates: 13g * Fat: 0.4g

Spicy Spinach Dumplings

Preparation Time: 10 minutes * Cooking Time: 10 minutes * Makes 10 pieces

Ingredients

2 teacups finely chopped spinach
1 chopped green chili
1 tablespoon gram flour (besan)
2 teaspoons whole wheat flour
2 teaspoons fresh curds (optional)
A pinch asafoetida
A pinch sugar
1 teaspoon oil
Salt to taste

Mix all the ingredients, using curds if the mixture is too dry for shaping

Shape into small flat rounds

Steam the rounds in a cooker for 5 to 7 minutes

- Serve Hot

Health Information: A light , vitamin rich snack for spinach lovers made using the calorie reducing steaming technique.

Per Paratha: Calories: 17 * Protein: 1g * Carbohydrates: 2g * Fat: 0.6g

Spicy Tomato Rasam

Preparation Time: 5 minutes * Cooking Time: 25 minutes * Makes 12 cups

Ingredients
For the Masala powder
1 teaspoon cumin seeds
1-1/2 teaspoons coriander seeds
8 peppercorns
Other Ingredients

1 kg tomatoes
3 tablespoons tamarind water
1 teaspoons lemon juice
2 pinches turmeric powder
½ teaspoon chilli powder
¼ teaspoon asafoetida
Salt to taste
For garnish

1 tablespoon chopped coriander
For the Masala Powder

Roast the cumin seeds, coriander seeds and peppercorns for 1 minute. Grind into a masala powder

How to Proceed

Cut the tomatoes in half and place in 8 glasses of boiling water

Add the remaining ingredients including the masala powder and boil for a further 10 minutes

Break the tomatoes with a spoon
Boil again for 10 minutes

- Garnish with chopped coriander and Serve hot.

Health Information: In this South Indian recipe, the spices help to increase flavour and decrease salt requirement. Tomatoes provide a lot of Vitamins A, C, and K.

Per Cup: Calories: 25 * Protein: 1g * Carbohydrates: 5g * Fat: 0.4g

Spinach and Vegetable Delight

Preparation time: 10 minutes * Cooking time: 10 minutes * Serves 6.

Ingredients

4 teacups chopped spinach
1 tablespoons gram (chana) dal 100 grams chopped mixed boiled vegetables (french beans, carrots, cauliflower, green peas)
1 chopped tomato

1 chopped onion 25 mm. Piece ginger, minced ½ teaspoon turmeric powder
1 teaspoon coriander powder
1 teaspoon chilli powder
2 teaspoon oil
Salt to taste

Soak the dal in water for 3 hours, Drain.

Heat the oil and fry the onion for 3 minutes.

Add the vegetables and tomato and fry again for 3 minutes.

Add the ginger, turmeric, coriander and chili powders and salt and mix well.

Add the soaked dal and cook for 2 minutes

Add the spinach and cook for 2 minutes while stirring continually.

Cook the mixture in a pressure cooker until 2 whistles.

Beat the mixture withy an egg-beater.

- Serve hot.

Health Information : This recipe contains an excellent combination of proteins from gram dal, the goodness of iron from spinach and the fibre and vitamins from other vegetables.

Per Serving: Calories 66 * Protein 4g * Carbohydrates 9g * Fat 2.4g.

Spinach Stuffing for Plain Parathas

Preparation Time: 10 minutes * Cooking Time: 5 minutes * For 12 Parathas

Ingredients

4 teacups finely chopped spinach
2 chopped onions
2 chopped green chilies
4 tablespoons crumbled paneer
2 teaspoons oil
Salt to taste

Heat the oil and fry the onions for ½ minutes. Add the green chilies and fry again for a few seconds

Add the spinach and cook for 2 minute
Drain the water, if any
Add the paneer and salt

Health Information: Spinach is a good source of folic acid, Vitamin A, iron and calcium and is good for growing children.

Per Paratha: Calories: 25, * Protein: 2g * Carbohydrates: 2.5g * Fat: 1g

Stuffed Bajra Roti

Preparation Time: 10 minutes * Cooking Time: 30 minutes * Makes 8 rotis

Ingredients

For the dough

2 teacups bajra flour

A pinch salt

To be mixed into a stuffing

½ teacup crumbled paneer
2 tablespoons chopped fenugreek (methi) leaves
1 chopped green chili
1 finely chopped large tomato
Salt to taste
For Serving

2 teaspoons butter (optional)
For the dough
Add salt and hot water to the bajra flour and make dough

Knead well, divide into 16 portions and roll out each portion into thin rotis

How to proceed

Spread a little stuffing on one roti. Then put another roti on top and press well so that it becomes one roti. Repeat for the remaining rotis and stuffing.

Cook each stuffed roti on a tawa (griddle) on both sides without oil.

- Serve hot. If you like, apply a little butter, before serving.

Health Information: Bajra is a coarse millet which has no gluten and can be eaten by people requiring gluten free diets. This roti is high in fibe and iron

Per Paratha: Calories: 115 * Protein: 7g * Carbohydrates: 18g * Fat: 1.4g

Suji Idli

Preparation Time: 10 minutes * Cooking Time: 25 minutes * Makes 70 small idlis

Ingredients How to ?
1 teacup semolina (suji)
1 teacup fresh curds
1 teaspoon fruit salt
1 teacup finely chopped cabbage
1 chopped onion
2 tablespoons chopped coriander a few curry leaves
2 to 3 finely chopped green chilies salt to taste

Roast the semolina on a tawa (griddle) without any oil until it becomes yellow or very light pink in colour

Mix the curds with the fruit salt and add the remaining ingredients to make a batter

Steam in a small idli mould for 10 minutes

- Serve hot

Health Information: Small finger snacks which are low in calories. Rich in Vitamins K, C and essential amino acids

Per Paratha: Calories: 8 * Protein: 0.5g * Carbohydrates: 2g * Fat: 0g

Tomato and Cauliflower Curry

Preparation time: 10 minutes * Cooking time: 30 minutes * Makes 6 cups.

Ingredients

½ kg. Tomatoes
¼ kg. Cauliflower
4 teaspoons gram flour (besan)
10 guar or clustered beans, cut into pieces

10 okra (ladies' fingers), cut into big pieces

2 tablespoons sliced white pumpkin (lauki)

2 slit green chilies
½ teaspoon mustard seeds

½ teaspoon cumin seeds a pinch asafetida

2 teaspoons oil
Salt to taste

Cook the tomatoes and cauliflower in 6 teacups of water until soft. Blend in a mixer.

Mix the gram flour with ¼ teacup of water and add to the mixture.

Add the remaining vegetables, green chilies, chili powder and salt and boil for 15 minutes.

Heat the oil and fry the mustard seeds and cumin seeds until they crackle. Add the asafetida.

Add to the mixture and boil again for 5 minutes.

- Serve hot.

Health Information: Rich in fibre, this recipe contains pumpkin and guar which add to the nutrient value. Guar has the effect of reducing blood sugar and may be used as an additive to flour for diabetics.

Per Serving: Calories 67 * Protein 3g * Carbohydrates 10g * Fat 2.4g

CHAPTER 9

HERBS & SPICES

History

Wars have been fought and countries discovered because of treasured spices. Marco Polo's stories of his trip to China in the late 1200s told of the spice trade in these then unknown lands and brought many Europeans in search of spices. In the 15th to 17th centuries the Spanish, English, Portuguese, and Dutch traders competed in the spice trade from the Far East. By the 1800s America was involved in the spice trade. America's first millionaires made their money in the spice trade. Many families in the colonies had their own herb gardens. Herbs and spices were also imported. These were used for cuisine specialties, as preservatives for the food supply, and for special medications. During the 1800s spices contained large amounts of fibrous or woody materials. Better processing techniques have done much to solve this problem. In the early 1900s many salesmen went from door-to-door selling spices; Golden Rule, Watkins, Raleigh, and McNess were some of the well-known brands.

Use of Herbs and Spices

The use of herbs and spices in cooking offers the chance to prepare exotic, gourmet dishes, or cultural meals and a way to cut or save calories and fat in cooking. Diet related diseases (heart disease, cancer, stroke, diabetes, and atherosclerosis) accounted for 66% of all deaths in Virginia in 1994. The cost for treatment of any one of these diseases averages $27,000 per person each year. Using herbs and spices can moderate dietary levels of fat, sugar and sodium. For example, removing a tablespoon of fat removes about 10 grams of fat and 100 calories - an amount which could represent a 10 pound weight loss in a year. The calories in herbs and spices are far less than in breadings, batters, gravies, sauces and fried foods. Cost savings are realized by reducing the number of ingredients in preparation and/or by the possibility of dressing up inexpensive foods for a special meal.

Many people are looking for flavors to substitute for salt or sodium. A teaspoon of salt has 2300 mg sodium - almost the amount recommended as the daily requirement. Many other condiments as well as packaged and processed foods contain around 1000 mg salt. Seasoning salts are regular salt with seasoning. A teaspoon of most herbs and spices contains few calories and little or no sodium. Herbs and spices add zest and flavor to unsalted foods.

Definitions of Herbs and Spices

Definitions of herbs and spices vary somewhat but can be identified as follows:

Herbs are leaves of low-growing shrubs. Examples are parsley, chives, marjoram, thyme, basil, caraway, dill, oregano, rosemary, savory, sage and celery leaves. These can be used fresh or dried. Dried forms may be whole, crushed, or ground. Many herbs can be grown in the United States in or out of doors.

Spices come from the bark (cinnamon), root (ginger, onion, garlic), buds (cloves, saffron), seeds (yellow mustard, poppy, sesame), berry (black pepper), or the fruit (allspice, paprika) of tropical plants and trees.

Many dehydrated vegetable seasonings are available. These include onion, garlic, sweet peppers, mint, mixed vegetables, and freeze-dried chives and shallots.

Condiments are usually a combination of herbs and spices blended in a liquid form. Examples are prepared mustard, catsup, Worcestershire sauce, tabasco sauce, and many of the steak sauces and specialty vinegars. Many of these contain sodium.

Seasoning blends are mixtures of spices and herbs. Check spice companies for exact mixtures. Some examples of seasoning blends are:

- Chili powder (red pepper, cumin, oregano, salt, and garlic powder)
- Curry powder (coriander, turmeric, cumin, fenugreek seed, white pepper, allspice, yellow mustard, red pepper, and ginger)
- Poultry seasoning (white pepper, sage, thyme, marjoram, savory, ginger, allspice, and nutmeg)
- Pumpkin pie spice (cinnamon, ginger, nutmeg, allspice, and cloves)

Storing Spices

Whole herbs and spices last much longer than crushed or ground forms. Many consumers prefer to buy the whole form and crush or grind as needed for greater freshness. Herbs and spices can be crushed with a mortar and pestle, by using a rolling pin with spices between two cloths, or by using the back of a spoon in a cup.

Check ground or crushed herbs and spices for freshness at least once a year. If no aroma is detected after crushing, the seasoning needs to be replaced. Mustard seed and poppy seed aromas will be difficult to detect. Buying the smaller size instead of the economy size container will save money if the large package is not used while it is still fresh.

1. Store away from moisture. Dampness causes caking and a loss of quality.
   Store in tightly covered, air tight container.

   Use clean, dry spoons for measuring.
2. Store in a cool place.
   Do not store in a window or in sunlight, or near heat sources such as the cooking areas or the dishwasher.

   In hot climates, store spices such as paprika, red pepper, and chili powder in the refrigerator to maintain quality.

Storage Life of Herbs and Spices
Seasoning Storage Time
Whole 2-5 years
Ground Spices 6 months-2 years
Leafy Herbs 3 months-2 years
Dehydrated Vegetables 6 months rice
Enhancing Sweet Flavors

Enhance flavor with sweet tasting spices instead of sugar: allspice, anise, cardamon, cinnamon, cloves, ginger, mace, nutmeg. Milk-Yogurt-Cheese: custards, puddings, sauces Meats: beef, fish, poultry, sauces, bean dishes Vegetables: beets, carrots, sweet potatoes, squash, pumpkin Fruits: fruit compote, baked fruit, spiced fruit Breads: gingerbread, sweet yeast breads, pumpkin bread, banana bread, rice or bread pudding.

Enhancing Savory Flavors

Seasoned salts (garlic salt) contain salt. Most meat sauces (steak sauce, soy sauce) are high in sodium.

Make yogurt-based spicy dressings to use with salads and fruit dishes. The following spices are good to use as a substitute for salt/sodium and fat: basil, bay leaf, celery seed, chili powder, cumin, curry powder, dill, marjoram, mustard, oregano, paprika, pepper, rosemary, sage, tarragon, thyme.

You can use these spices with fondue, cheese spread, chowder, meats, souffl», curried dishes, beans and soups, salads, greens, tomatoes/juice, pasta salads, specialty breads, and rice.

The Art of Seasoning

The art of using herbs and spices is learning how much to add and how to combine flavors. Several guidelines suggest amounts to use in developing recipes: Use strong, pungent spices such as red pepper in small amounts. More delicate seasoning can be used in greater amounts without ruining the final product. Although the herb or spice should enhance and not overpower the flavor, cultural preferences will influence your decision.

Start with a tested recipe. After it has been prepared, decide if more or less seasoning is needed for the next time. Spice and herb companies recommend about ¼ teaspoon (a pinch) of spice per pound of meat or pint of liquid when creating recipes. Only use 1/8 teaspoon of stronger seasonings such as red pepper and garlic. Remember, it is easier to add more than to try to compensate for too much.

More than one herb or spice can be used in a recipe. When creating a recipe, start by using only one or two choices. As you gain experience in cooking with herbs and spices, taste will tell if others might be added.

Herb Bread

Many cultural specialties feature yeast breads and quick breads using a variety of spices and herbs.

Add the following ingredients per pound (3 to 4 cups flour) of yeast dough. 1 tsp. sage, 2 tsp. caraway seed, and 1 ½ tsp. nutmeg

1 ½ Tbsp. dill seed or 1 ½ Tbsp. caraway seed and 1/8 cup instant minced onion

½ tsp. sage, ½ tsp. thyme, and ½ tsp. marjoram

Herb Vinegar Dressings

Use with vegetable salads or cooked vegetables.

1/8 tsp. ground black pepper, 1 tsp. dry mustard, ½ tsp. paprika, ¾ tsp. garlic powder, 1 Tbsp. finely chopped chives, 3 Tbsp. cider vinegar, ½ cup vegetable oil, 2 Tbsp. pickle relish, 2 Tbsp. lemon juice. Yield: ¾ to 1 cup

¾ cup tomato juice, 2 Tbsp. lemon juice, 2 Tbsp. instant minced onion, 1 Tbsp. basil leaves crushed, ¼ tsp. garlic powder, 1/8 tsp. ground cumin seed, 1/8 tsp. ground red pepper. Yield: ¾ to 1 cup.

Adding Spices to a Recipe

Whole Spices and Herbs

Tie herbs and spices in a cheesecloth, nylon net or muslin bag, or place them in a tea ring. The bag or ring is easy to remove to stop the seasoning process. Particles that may cause difficulty in chewing or swallowing also can be removed.

Add whole herbs and spices at the start of cooking in recipes that will cook for an hour or longer. Examples are soups and stews.

Many herbal and spiced teas can be made using whole herbs and spices.

Flavoring seeds can be toasted briefly in the oven or on top of the stove to enhance flavor. Whole herbs are usually crumbled and added near the end of cooking.

Crushed and Ground Herbs and Spices

Add about 15 minutes before the end of cooking. The flavors in crushed or ground spices are released quickly.

Crushing or grinding whole spices and herbs provides more flavor than the whole form. Ground black pepper in a pepper shaker does not have the zest of freshly ground pepper. Grinding pepper from the pepper corn provides more flavor.

For cold salad dressings, mix herbs and/or spices with vinegar for several hours before adding oil in order to develop the flavor.

Be Creative

Be both a scientist and an artist as you learn to cook with spices. Start with several herbs and spices, learning to know the flavoring and how it complements different dishes. Look for new ideas by checking labels on spice packages and by collecting recipes on regional or other specialty dishes.

Sources of Vitamin A

Fruits	% Vitamin A
Apricot	45 %
Cantaloupe	100 %
Dried apricots	50 %
Mango	40 %
Watermelon	20 %

Vegetables	**% Vitamin A**
Carrot	270 %
Collards	50 %
Hot chili peppers	80 %
Leaf Lettuce	40 %
Mustard Greens	90 %
Romaine Lettuce	20 %
Spinach	70 %
Sweet Potato	440 %
Tomato	20 %

Remember: Eat at least one vitamin A rich fruit or vegetable, such as cantaloupe, carrots, sweet potato, spinach, or broccoli every day.

Sources of Vitamin C

Our list shows fruits and vegetables which are high in vitamin C. That means they contain at least 20% of the daily value of vitamin C in one serving. Look through the list and find your favorites! Eat at least one fruit or vegetable high in vitamin C every day.

Fruits	% Vitamin C
Apricot	20 %
Blackberries	50 %
Cantaloupe	80 %
Carambola	30 %
Gooseberries	60 %
Grapefruit	110 %
Grapes	25 %
Honeydew Melon	45 %
Kiwifruit	240 %
Lemon	40 %
Lime	35 %
Orange	130 %
Papaya	150 %
Pineapple	25 %
Plum	20 %
Pricklypear	25 %
Pummelo	130 %
Raspberries	40 %
Strawberries	160 %
Tangerine	50 %
Watermelon	25 %

Remember: Eat at least one vitamin C rich fruit or vegetable, such as grapefruit, oranges, green pepper, or cauliflower every day.

High Sources of Fiber

High sources provide at least 20% (5 grams) of the daily value of fiber per serving.

Fruits	% Fiber
Apple	20 %
Blackberries	22 %
Grapefruit	24 %
Orange	28 %
Raspberries	32 %
Vegetables	% Fiber
Broccoli	20 %

Good Sources of Fiber

Good sources provide at least 10% (2.5 grams) of the daily value of fiber per serving.

Fruits	% Fiber
Avocado	12 %
Banana	16 %
Blueberries	14 %
Cherries	12 %
Dates	12 %
Dried Figs	12 %
Figs	16 %
Kiwifruit	16 %
Papaya	10 %
Pear	16 %
Prunes	12 %
Strawberries	16 %
Tangerine	12 %

Vegetables	% Fiber
Artichoke	11 %
Brussels Sprouts	12 %
Corn	12 %
Green beans	12 %
Onion	12 %
Potato	12 %
Spinach	19 %
Sweet Potato	16 %

Remember: Eat at least one high fiber fruit or vegetable, such as apples, grapefruit, or broccoli every day.

Importance of Folate

Folate has been in the news lately because it is linked to the prevention of birth defects (such as spina bifida), heart attacks, stroke and colorectal cancer. Folate, a B Vitamin, is also referred to as folic acid or folacin.

All adult men and women need to 400 micrograms of folate in their diet each day. However, most Americans do not eat enough folate. The good news is that by eating at least 5 servings of fruits and vegetables a day and eating dried peas and beans several times a week you can ensure that your diet contains adequate folate for good health.

Our list shows fruits and vegetables which are good or high sources of folate. Look though the list and find your favorites. Eat at least one fruit or vegetable that is a good or high source of folate every day.

Sources of Folate

High sources provide at least 20% (80 micrograms) of the daily value of folate per serving.

Black-eye Peas
Broccoli
Kidney Beans
Lentils
Mustard Greens
Spinach
Split Peas
Strawberries
Turnip Greens
White Beans

Good sources provide at least 10% (40 micrograms) of the daily value of folate per serving.

Beets
Cabbage
Cauliflower
Green Cauliflower
Grapefruit Juice
Orange
Orange Juice
Papaya
Red Bell Pepper

Sweet Potato

Remember: Eat at least one fruit or vegetable that is a good or high source of folate every day.

Are tomatoes fruits or vegetables?

Plant scientists say tomatoes are fruits because they contain seeds. However, most nutritionists think of tomatoes as vegetables because they contain so few calories compared to other fruits. For example, a medium apple contains about 80 calories while a medium tomato contains only 20 calories.

Tomatoes aren't the only fruit most people think of as vegetables. Cucumbers, peppers, eggplant and squash are also considered fruit because they contain seeds. While this is a very simple explanation of the differences between fruits and vegetables, in most cases it works. Think about foods that contain seeds; most are considered fruits by plant scientists. Defining vegetables so simply is not that easy. Vegetables can be edible roots (e.g. carrots), tubers (e.g. potatoes), stems (e.g. celery), flowers (e.g. broccoli) or leaves (e.g. lettuce).

Is it dangerous to drink grapefruit juice when taking medication?

Both grapefruit and grapefruit juice may interfere with the metabolism of certain medications. The most common result is higher than expected levels of the medication in the body. These increased levels can result in dangerous side effects.

The effect of grapefruit products on the metabolism of certain medications can last for more than 24 hours, so taking the medication at another time is not advised. The best way to avoid the dangerous effects of grapefruit products is to avoid the products altogether when taking medications affected by grapefruit products.

Be sure to discuss any concerns about combining grapefruit products with medications you may be taking with your pharmacist and physician.

What's the difference between sweet potatoes and yams?

There are many differences between sweet potatoes and yams. Sweet potatoes are roots of a vine in the morning glory family. Yams are tubers of a tropical vine. Sweet potatoes are rich in vitamin A while yams contain no vitamin A.

To make this issue more confusing, there are two types of sweet potatoes. The paler-skinned sweet potato has a thin, light yellow skin with pale yellow flesh, which is not sweet and has a dry, crumbly texture similar to a white baking potato. The darker-skinned variety (which is most often called "yam" in error) has a thicker, dark orange skin with a vivid orange, sweet flesh with a moist texture. U.S. supermarkets tend to carry both types of sweet potatoes but incorrectly label the darker-skinned variety "yams."

True yams are rarely available in U.S. markets. If you find yams, they will most likely be sold in chunks sealed in plastic wrap, since they grow up to 7 feet in length and weigh up to 150 pounds! The yam tuber has a brown or black skin, which resembles the bark of a tree, and off-white, purple or red flesh, depending on the variety.

Where do baby carrots come from?

Baby carrots are cut from bigger carrots. A special variety of carrot called "caropak carrots" are grown for mini-peeled carrots. Caropak carrots are grown close together, which results in thinner, more tender carrots. After harvesting, the carrots are washed in chlorinated water, just like our drinking water, and cleaned to remove dirt and mud. They are then sorted to separate out those that are too large or too small. The carrots selected to become mini-peeled are then cut into 2" lengths and the skin is peeled. A final polishing process rounds their corners. Then they are packaged in 1 ounce, ½ pound, 1 pound or 5 pound bags.

Why do apples turn brown when cut?

Cut apples turn brown because of a reaction called oxidation. Oxygen in the air reacts with a natural substance in apples called phenolase and turns the cut surface brown. Mild acids like lemon juice can stop this reaction; tossing cut apple chunks with a little bit of lemon juice will keep the apples from turning brown.

Research on Fruits, Vegetables and Health

Researchers are continually investigating the numerous health-protecting properties of the phytochemicals in fruits and vegetables. (Phytochemicals are substances produced by plants that help to protect them from insects, diseases and other threats to their health. These same substances help to protect human health.) While more than 4000 phytochemicals have been identified, fewer than 200 phytochemicals have been studied extensively. Summaries of recently published studies examining the health benefits of eating fruits and vegetables are presented here.

An Apple A Day May Keep the Heart and Lung Specialists Away

Researchers at the University of California Davis Medical School studied how eating apples and drinking apple juice every day affects heart disease risk. The 12-week study showed that by simply including apples in the diet (and without making any other dietary changes), study participants were able to reduce their risk of heart disease. Apples contain a variety of antioxidant phytochemicals that decrease LDL oxidation. Oxidized LDL cholesterol is more likely to build up in arteries, a process that can cause heart attacks and stroke.

Researchers from the University of Nottingham, located in the United Kingdom, recently reported that people who eat five or more apples a week have better lung function and lower risk of asthma and other respiratory disease compared to people who rarely eat apples. Their findings were based on a 10-year study involving 2,633 people examining relationships between diet and respiratory health. The researchers suspect that antioxidants in apples lead to these health benefits. In 1997 Finnish researchers reported that the antioxidant flavonoids may reduce the risk of lung cancer.

CHAPTER 10

ALERT ON COMMON DISORDERS

Carotenoids and Cancer

Carrots and other orange vegetables like squash and sweet potato and dark green vegetables like broccoli and spinach contain phytochemicals called carotenoids. The Nurses' Health Study showed that women who eat the most carotenoid-rich vegetables have the lowest risk of breast cancer. Researchers report that raw vegetables contain the highest amounts of carotenoids, which are damaged by the heat of cooking.

The Cruciferous Crusaders

Cruciferous vegetables include bok choy, broccoli, brussels sprouts, cabbage, cauliflower, collard greens, rutabaga and turnips. Researchers from the Fred Hutchinson Cancer Research Center in Seattle reported in 2000 that men who eat at least 1.5 cups of cruciferous vegetables a week can reduce their prostate cancer risk by more than 40 percent. Researchers speculate that phytochemicals in cruciferous vegetables called isothiocyanates help the body produce enzymes that destroy cancer-causing compounds.

What is the best thing to do nutritionally if you have abdominal pain?

Sometimes it is best to rest the pancreas and limit your food intake. If you are experiencing a flare, your doctor may even recommend no food for a day or two. If you can tolerate food, low fat, low protein foods may be better tolerated as they tend to stimulate the pancreas the least. Avoid high fat and heavily spiced foods. If you notice a particular food causes pain, avoid it. A diet of only clear liquids can be followed when pain is severe. Clear liquids include apple, cranberry and grape juice, gelatin and broth. The clear liquid diet, however, is not nutritionally complete and the diet should be advanced as soon as additional food is tolerated.

What can be done for nutrition when there is nausea and vomiting?

The following suggestions may help you maintain or increase your intake while minimizing nausea and vomiting:

- Avoid foods with high fat content (such as greasy or fried foods).
- Avoid coffee, tea, and alcohol. Cool, clear liquids are often better tolerated. Try broth, flavored gelatin, carbonated beverages, popsicles, or apple juice. Drink small amounts every hour, especially if you are vomiting.
- Eat smaller portions more often during the day. Eating small amounts every 1-2 hours may be helpful.
- Don't drink liquids with your meals. It is best to drink fluids 45-60 minutes before or after meals.
- Avoid spicy foods. Bland foods may be better tolerated.
- Foods that are cold or warm may be easier to tolerate than hot foods.
- Let someone else do the cooking. The odor of foods may make you feel worse.

How can someone with pancreatitis or other pancreatic diseases go out to a restaurant?

Most restaurants are more than willing to accomodate special requests. When ordering in a restaurant, request a very low fat meal and explain to the server that there is a medical reason for the request. Most restaurants will steam fish and vegetables or grill a piece of chicken. Many restaurants are happy to take on the challenge and will produce a truly delicious meal for you.

Stomach Ulcers

Duodenal ulcers often occur between the ages of 30 and 50, and are twice as common among men. Stomach ulcers are more common after the age of 60 and are more commonly seen in women.

What Is An Ulcer?

An ulcer is a focal area of the stomach or duodenum that has been destroyed by digestive juices and stomach acid. Most ulcers are no larger than a pencil eraser, but they can cause tremendous discomfort and pain.

What Are The Symptoms Of Ulcers?

The most common symptom of an ulcer is a gnawing or burning pain in the abdomen located between the navel and the bottom of the breastbone. The pain often occurs between meals and sometimes awakens people from sleep. Pain may last minutes to hours and is often relived by eating and taking antacids. Less common symptoms of an ulcer include nausea, vomiting and loss of appetite and weight.

What Causes Ulcers?

In the past, ulcers were incorrectly thought to be caused by stress. Doctors now know that there are two major causes of ulcers. Most often patients are infected with the bacteria Helicobacter pylori (H. pylori). Others who develop ulcers are regular users of pain medications called nonsteroidal anti-inflammatory drugs (NSAIDS), which include common products like aspirin and ibuprofen. The use of antibiotics to fight the H. pylori infection is a major scientific advance. Studies now show that antibiotics can permanently cure 80-90 percent of peptic ulcers. Blocking stomach acid remains very important in the initial healing of an ulcer.

Helicobacter Pylori

The largest number of ulcers arise because of the presence of Helicobacter pylori. Because H. pylori exists in the stomachs of some people who do not develop ulcers, most scientists now believe that ulcers occur in persons who have a combination of a genetic predisposition, plus the presence of the bacteria, Helicobacter pylori.

Use Of Nonsteroidal Anti-Inflammatory Drugs (NSAIDS)

The second major cause for ulcers is irritation of the stomach arising from regular use of nonsteroidal anti-inflammatory drugs. NSAID-induced gastrointestinal side effects can best be avoided by using alternative therapy whenever possible. Low-dose corticosteroids or supportive drugs such as acetaminophen are alternatives to NSAIDS to consider. Four grams per day of acetaminophen has been shown to be comparable to analgesic and anti-inflammatory doses of ibuprofen for osteoarthritis pain and is not associated with an increased risk of gastrointestinal side effects.

If you are taking over-the-counter pain medications on a regular basis, you will want to talk with your physician about the potential for ulcers and other GI side effects. Your doctor may recommend a change in the medication you are using, that you take some other medication in conjunction with your pain medication. These could range from use of antacids or a prescription product (such as misoprostol) in conjunction with your pain medication.

What Are The Complications Of Ulcers?

- Bleeding. Bleeding from an ulcer can occur in the stomach or the duodenum and is sometimes the only sign of an ulcer. Bleeding from an ulcer may be slow, causing anemia and fatigue. More rapid bleeding can cause bowel movements to become sticky and tarry black or even bloody. Bleeding ulcers may cause nausea and vomiting of acidified blood that looks like "old coffee grounds."
- Perforation. When ulcers are left untreated digestive juices and stomach acid can literally eat a hole in the intestinal lining. Bacteria, food and digestive juices can spill into the abdominal cavity causing sudden, intense pain that requires hospitalization, and often surgery.
- Obstruction. Chronic inflammation from an ulcer can cause swelling and scarring to occur. Over time scarring may close the outlet of the stomach, preventing food to pass and causing vomiting and weight loss.

How Are Ulcers Diagnosed?

Most doctors recommend that a test be performed to evaluate for the presence of an ulcer if symptoms are not improved after 2 weeks of treatment with an acid blocking medicine (citnetidine, ranitidine, famotidine, omeprazole or lansaprazole etc.). The two tests most commonly used to evaluate for ulcer are an X-ray known as an Upper GI Series (UGI), and a procedure called an Endoscopy (EGD). An UGI series is an X-ray test where you are given a chalky material to drink while X-rays are taken to outline the anatomy of the digestive tract. An EGD is a test that involves insertion of a small lighted flexible tube through the mouth into the esophagus and stomach to examine for abnormalities. The test is usually performed using medicines to sedate you. During the test biopsies of tissue can be taken for examination. A biopsy will not cause any pain or discomfort and is usually only the size of a match head.

Tests For Helicobacter Pylori

There are several tests available to your doctor to evaluate for the presence of the bacteria, H. pylori. Samples of blood can be examined for evidence of antibodies to the bacteria; a breath test can be examined for by-products from the bacteria; or biopsies from the stomach can be examined.

How Are Ulcers Treated?

In the past, doctors advised patients to avoid spicy, fatty and acidic foods. We now know that diet has little to do with ulcer healing. Doctors now recommend that patients with ulcers only avoid foods that worsen their symptoms. Ulcer patients who smoke cigarettes should stop. Smoking has been shown to inhibit ulcer healing and is linked to ulcer recurrence. In general, ulcer patients should not take NSAIDS like aspirin or ibuprofen.

When Is Surgery Necessary?

Most ulcers can be healed with medications. When an ulcer fails to heal or if complications of bleeding, perforation or obstruction develop, surgery is often necessary.

Peptic Ulcer

A peptic ulcer is a sore on the lining of the stomach or duodenum, which is the beginning of the small intestine. Peptic ulcers are common: one in every 10 Americans develops an ulcer at some time in his or her life. The main cause of peptic ulcer is bacterial infection, but some ulcers are caused by long-term use of nonsteroidal anti-inflammatory agents (NSAIDs), like aspirin and ibuprofen. In a few cases, cancerous tumors in the stomach or pancreas can cause ulcers. Peptic ulcers are not caused by spicy food or stress.

What Is H. pylori?

Helicobacter pylori (H. pylori) is a type of bacteria. Researchers recently discovered that H. pylori causes almost all peptic ulcers, accounting for 80 percent of stomach ulcers and more than 90 percent of duodenal ulcers. H. pylori infection is common in the United States: about 20 percent of people under 40 and half of people over 60 are infected with it. Most infected people, however, do not develop ulcers. Why H. pylori doesn't cause ulcers in every infected person is unknown. Most likely, infection depends on characteristics of the infected person, the type of H. pylori, and other factors yet to be discovered.

Researchers are not certain how people become infected with H. pylori, but they think it may be through food or water.

Researchers have found H. pylori in some infected people's saliva, so the bacteria may also spread through mouth-to-mouth contact such as kissing.

How Does H. pylori Cause A Peptic Ulcer?

H. pylori weakens the protective mucous coating of the stomach and duodenum, which allows acid to get through to the sensitive lining beneath. Both the acid and the bacteria irritate the lining and cause a sore, or ulcer. H. pylori is able to survive in stomach acid because it secretes enzymes that neutralize the acid. This mechanism allows H. pylori to make its way to the "safe" area—the protective mucous lining. Once there, the bacterium's spiral shape helps it burrow through the mucous lining.

What Are The Symptoms Of An Ulcer?

Pain is the most common symptom. The pain usually:

- Is a dull, gnawing ache.
- Comes and goes for several days or weeks.
- Occurs 2 to 3 hours after a meal.
- Occurs in the middle of the night (when the stomach is empty).
- Is relieved by food.

Other symptoms include:

- Weight loss.
- Poor appetite.
- Bloating.

- Burping.
- Nausea.
- Vomiting.

Some people experience only very mild symptoms, or none at all.

Emergency Symptoms

If you have any of these symptoms, call your doctor right away:

- Sharp, sudden, persistent stomach pain.
- Bloody or black stools.
- Bloody vomit or vomit that looks like coffee grounds.

They could be signs of a serious problem, such as:

- Perforation—when the ulcer burrows through the stomach or duodenal wall.
- Bleeding—when acid or the ulcer breaks a blood vessel.
- Obstruction—when the ulcer blocks the path of food trying to leave the stomach.

How Is An H. pylori-related Ulcer Diagnosed?

Diagnosing An Ulcer

To see if symptoms are caused by an ulcer, the doctor may do an upper gastrointestinal (GI) series or an endoscopy. An upper GI series is an x-ray of the esophagus, stomach, and duodenum. The patient drinks a chalky liquid called barium to make these organs and any ulcers show up more clearly on the x-ray.

An endoscopy is an exam with an endoscope, a thin, lighted tube with a tiny camera on the end. The patient is lightly sedated, and the doctor carefully eases the endoscope through the patient's mouth and down the throat to the stomach and duodenum. This allows the doctor to see the lining of the esophagus, stomach, and duodenum. The doctor can use the endoscope to take photos of ulcers or remove a tiny piece of tissue to view under a microscope.

Diagnosing H. pylori

If an ulcer is found, the doctor will test the patient for H. pylori. This test is important because treatment for an ulcer caused by H. pylori is different from that for an ulcer caused by NSAIDs.

H. pylori is diagnosed through blood, breath, and tissue tests. Blood tests are most common. They detect antibodies to H. pylori bacteria. Blood is taken at the doctor's office through a finger stick.

Breath tests are mainly used after treatment to see if treatment worked, but they can be used in diagnosis, too. The test is called a urea breath test.

In the doctor's office, the patient drinks a solution of urea that contains a special carbon atom. If H. pylori is present, it breaks down the urea, releasing the carbon. The blood carries the carbon to the lungs, where the patient exhales it. The breath test is 96 percent to 98 percent accurate.

Tissue tests are usually done using tissue removed with the endoscope. There are three types:

- The rapid urease test detects the enzyme urease, which is produced by H. pylori.
- A histology test allows the doctor to find and examine the actual bacteria.
- A culture test involves allowing H. pylori to grow in the tissue sample.

How Are H. pylori Peptic Ulcers Treated?

H. pylori peptic ulcers are treated with drugs to kill the bacteria, to reduce stomach acid, and to protect the stomach lining. Antibiotics are used to kill the bacteria. Two types of acid-suppressing drugs might be used: H2-blockers and proton pump inhibitors.

H2-blockers work by blocking histamine, which stimulates acid secretion. They help reduce ulcer pain after a few weeks. Proton pump inhibitors suppress acid production by halting the mechanism that pumps the acid into the stomach. H2-blockers and proton pump inhibitors have been prescribed alone for years as treatments for ulcers. But used alone, these drugs do not eradicate H. pylori, and therefore do not cure H. pylori-related ulcers. Bismuth subsalicylate, a component of Pepto-Bismol, is used to protect the stomach lining from acid. It also kills H. pylori. Treatment usually involves a combination of antibiotics, acid suppressors, and stomach protectors.

- Antibiotics: metronidazole, tetracycline, clarithromycin,amoxicillin.
- H2-blockers: cimetidine, ranitidine, famotidine, nizatidine.
- Proton pump inhibitors: omeprazole, lansoprazole.
- Stomach-lining protector: bismuth subsalicylate.

At this time, the most proven effective treatment is a 2-week course of treatment called triple therapy. It involves taking two antibiotics to kill the bacteria and either an acid suppressor or stomach lining shield. Two-week triple therapy reduces ulcer symptoms, kills the bacteria, and prevents ulcer recurrence in more than 90 percent of patients.

Unfortunately, patients may find triple therapy complicated because it involves taking as many as 20 pills a day. Also, the antibiotics used in triple therapy may cause mild side effects such as nausea, vomiting, diarrhea, dark stools, metallic taste in the mouth, dizziness, headache, and yeast infections in women. (Most side effects can be treated with medication withdrawal.) Nevertheless, recent studies show that 2 weeks of triple therapy is ideal.

Early results of studies in other countries suggest that 1 week of triple therapy may be as effective as the 2-week therapy, with fewer side effects.

Another option is 2 weeks of dual therapy. Dual therapy involves two drugs: one antibiotic and one acid suppressor. It is not as effective as triple therapy.

Two weeks of quadruple therapy, which uses two antibiotics, an acid suppressor, and a stomach lining shield, looks promising in research studies. It is also called bismuth triple therapy.

After Treatment

To be sure that treatment has killed all H. pylori, the doctor will do a follow-up endoscopy or breath test 6 to 12 months after treatment to check for the bacterium.

Can H. pylori Infection Be Prevented?

No one knows for sure how H. pylori spreads, so prevention is difficult. Researchers are trying to develop a vaccine to prevent infection.

Why Don't All Doctors Automatically Check for H. pylori?

Changing medical belief and practice takes time. For nearly 100 years, scientists and doctors thought that ulcers were caused by stress, spicy food, and alcohol. Treatment involved bed rest and a bland diet. Later, researchers added stomach acid to the list of causes and began treating ulcers with antacids.

Since H. pylori was discovered in 1982, studies conducted around the world have shown that using antibiotics to destroy H. pylori cured peptic ulcers. The National Institutes of Health released a consensus statement in 1994 confirming that H. pylori causes peptic ulcers. Despite the evidence, however, the medical community continues to debate H. pylori's role in peptic ulcers. If you have a peptic ulcer and have not been tested for H. pylori infection, talk to your doctor.

Points To Remember

- A peptic ulcer is a sore in the lining of the stomach or duodenum.
- Most peptic ulcers are caused by the H. pylori bacterium. None are caused by spicy food or stress.
- H. pylori may be transmitted from person to person through contaminated food and water.
- Always wash your hands after using the bathroom and before eating.
- Antibiotics are the most effective treatment for H. pylori peptic ulcers.

Constipation

Definition & Causes Of Constipation

Constipation is passage of small amounts of hard, dry bowel movements, usually fewer than three times a week. People who are constipated may find it difficult and painful to have a bowel movement. Other symptoms of constipation include feeling bloated, uncomfortable, and sluggish.

Many people think they are constipated when, in fact, their bowel movements are regular. For example, some people believe they are constipated, or irregular, if they do not have a bowel movement every day. However, there is no right number of daily or weekly bowel movements. Normal may be three times a day or three times a week depending on the person. In addition, some people naturally have firmer stools than others.

At one time or another almost everyone gets constipated. Poor diet and lack of exercise are usually the causes. In most cases, constipation is temporary and not serious. Understanding causes, prevention, and treatment will help most people find relief.

Who Gets Constipated?

According to the 1991 National Health Interview Survey, about 4.5 million people in the United States say they are constipated most or all of the time. Those reporting constipation most often are women, children, and adults age 65 and over. Pregnant women also complain of constipation, and it is a common problem following childbirth or surgery.

Constipation is the most common gastrointestinal complaint in the United States, resulting in about 2 million annual visits to the doctor. However, most people treat themselves without seeking medical help.

What Causes Constipation?

To understand constipation, it helps to know how the colon (large intestine) works. As food moves through it, the colon absorbs water while forming waste products, or stool. Muscle contractions in the colon push the stool toward the rectum. By the time stool reaches the rectum, it is solid because most of the water has been absorbed.

The hard and dry stools of constipation occur when the colon absorbs too much water. This happens because the colon's muscle contractions are slow or sluggish, causing the stool to move through the colon too slowly.

Common Causes Of Constipation

- Not enough fiber in diet.
- Not enough liquids.
- Lack of exercise.
- Medications.
- Irritable bowel syndrome.

- Changes in life or routine such as pregnancy, older age, and travel.
- Abuse of laxatives.
- Ignoring the urge to have a bowel movement.
- Specific diseases such as multiple sclerosis and lupus.
- Problems with the colon and rectum.
- Problems with intestinal function (Chronic idiopathic constipation.)

Diet

The most common cause of constipation is a diet low in fiber found in vegetables, fruits, and whole grains and high in fats found in cheese, eggs, and meats. People who eat plenty of high-fiber foods are less likely to become constipated.

Fiber—soluble and insoluble—is the part of fruits, vegetables, and grains that the body cannot digest. Soluble fiber dissolves easily in water and takes on a soft, gel-like texture in the intestines. Insoluble fiber passes almost unchanged through the intestines. The bulk and soft texture of fiber help prevent hard, dry stools that are difficult to pass.

On average, Americans eat about 5 to 20 grams of fiber daily, short of the 20 to 35 grams recommended by the American Dietetic Association. Both children and adults eat too many refined and processed foods in which the natural fiber is removed.

A low-fiber diet also plays a key role in constipation among older adults. They often lack interest in eating and may choose fast foods low in fiber. In addition, loss of teeth may force older people to eat soft foods that are processed and low in fiber.

Not Enough Liquids

Liquids like water and juice add fluid to the colon and bulk to stools, making bowel movements softer and easier to pass. People who have problems with constipation should drink enough of these liquids every day, about eight 8-ounce glasses. Other liquids, like coffee and soft drinks, that contain caffeine seem to have a dehydrating effect.

Lack Of Exercise

Lack of exercise can lead to constipation, although doctors do not know precisely why. For example, constipation often occurs after an accident or during an illness when one must stay in bed and cannot exercise.

Medications

Pain medications (especially narcotics), antacids that contain aluminum, antispasmodics, antidepressants, iron supplements, diuretics, and anticonvulsants for epilepsy can slow passage of bowel movements.

Irritable Bowel Syndrome (IBS)

Some people with IBS, also known as spastic colon, have spasms in the colon that affect bowel movements. Constipation and diarrhea often alternate, and abdominal cramping, gassiness, and bloating are other common complaints. Although IBS can produce lifelong symptoms, it is not a life-threatening condition. It often worsens with stress, but there is no specific cause or anything unusual that the doctor can see in the colon.

Changes In Life Or Routine

During pregnancy, women may be constipated because of hormonal changes or because the heavy uterus compresses the intestine. Aging may also affect bowel regularity because a slower metabolism results in less intestinal activity and muscle tone. In addition, people often become constipated when traveling because their normal diet and daily routines are disrupted.

Abuse Of Laxatives

Myths about constipation have led to a serious abuse of laxatives. This is common among older adults who are preoccupied with having a daily bowel movement.

Laxatives usually are not necessary and can be habit-forming. The colon begins to rely on laxatives to bring on bowel movements. Over time, laxatives can damage nerve cells in the colon and interfere with the colon's natural ability to contract. For the same reason, regular use of enemas can also lead to a loss of normal bowel function.

Ignoring The Urge To Have A Bowel Movement

People who ignore the urge to have a bowel movement may eventually stop feeling the urge, which can lead to constipation. Some people delay having a bowel movement because they do not want to use toilets outside the home. Others ignore the urge because of emotional stress or because they are too busy. Children may postpone having a bowel movement because of stressful toilet training or because they do not want to interrupt their play.

Specific Diseases

Diseases that cause constipation include neurological disorders, metabolic and endocrine disorders, and systemic conditions that affect organ systems. These disorders can slow the movement of stool through the colon, rectum, or anus.

Diseases That Cause Constipation

Neurological disorders that may cause constipation include:

- Multiple sclerosis.
- Parkinson's disease.
- Chronic idiopathic intestinal pseudo-obstruction.
- Stroke.
- Spinal cord injuries.

Metabolic and endocrine conditions include:

- Diabetes.
- Underactive or overactive thyroid gland.
- Uremia.

Systemic disorders include:

- Amyloidosis.
- Lupus.
- Scleroderma.

Problems With The Colon & Rectum

Intestinal obstruction, scar tissue (adhesions), diverticulosis, tumors, colorectal stricture, Hirschsprung's disease, or cancer can compress, squeeze, or narrow the intestine and rectum and cause constipation.

Problems With Intestinal Function (Chronic Idiopathic Constipation)

Also known as functional constipation, chronic idiopathic (of unknown origin) constipation is rare. However, some people are chronically constipated and do not respond to standard treatment. This chronic constipation may be related to multiple problems with hormonal control or with nerves and muscles in the colon, rectum, or anus. Functional constipation occurs in both children and adults and is most common in women.

Colonic inertia and delayed transit are two types of functional constipation caused by decreased muscle activity in the colon. These syndromes may affect the entire colon or may be confined to the left or lower (sigmoid) colon.

Functional constipation that stems from abnormalities in the structure of the anus and rectum is known as anorectal dysfunction, or anismus. These abnormalities result in an inability to relax the rectal and anal muscles that allow stool to exit.

What Diagnostic Tests Are Used For Consitipation?

Most people do not need extensive testing and can be treated with changes in diet and exercise for their constipation. For example, in young people with mild symptoms, a medical history and physical examination may be all the doctor needs to suggest successful treatment. The tests the doctor performs depends on the duration and severity of the constipation, the person's age, and whether there is blood in stools, recent changes in bowel movements, or weight loss.

Medical History

The doctor may ask a patient to describe his or her constipation, including duration of symptoms, frequency of bowel movements, consistency of stools, presence of blood in the stool, and toilet habits (how often and where one has bowel movements). Recording eating habits, medication, and level of physical activity or exercise also helps the doctor determine the cause of constipation.

Physical Examination

A physical exam may include a digital rectal exam with a gloved, lubricated finger to evaluate the tone of the muscle that closes off the anus (anal sphincter) and to detect tenderness, obstruction, or blood. In some cases, blood and thyroid tests may be necessary.

Extensive testing usually is reserved for people with severe symptoms, for those with sudden changes in number and consistency of bowel movements or blood in the stool, and for older adults. Because of an increased risk of colorectal cancer in older adults, the doctor may use these tests to rule out a diagnosis of cancer:

- Barium enema x-ray.
- Sigmoidoscopy or colonoscopy.
- Colorectal transit study.
- Anorectal function tests.

Barium Enema X-Ray

A barium enema x-ray involves viewing the rectum, colon, and lower part of the small intestine to locate any problems. This part of the digestive tract is known as the bowel. This test may show intestinal obstruction and Hirschsprung's disease, a lack of nerves within the colon.

The night before the test, bowel cleansing, also called bowel prep, is necessary to clear the lower digestive tract. The patient drinks 8 ounces of a special liquid every 15 minutes for about 4 hours. This liquid flushes out the bowel. A clean bowel is important, because even a small amount of stool in the colon can hide details and result in an inaccurate exam.

Because the colon does not show up well on an x-ray, the doctor fills the organs with a barium enema, a chalky liquid to make the area visible. Once the mixture coats the organs, x-rays are taken that reveal their shape and condition. The patient may feel some abdominal cramping when the barium fills the colon, but usually feels little discomfort after the procedure. Stools may be a whitish color for a few days after the exam.

Sigmoidoscopy Or Colonoscopy

An examination of the rectum and lower colon (sigmoid) is called a sigmoidoscopy. An examination of the rectum and entire colon is called a colonoscopy.

The night before a sigmoidoscopy, the patient usually has a liquid dinner and takes an enema at bedtime. A light breakfast and a cleansing enema an hour before the test may also be necessary.

To perform a sigmoidoscopy, the doctor uses a long, flexible tube with a light on the end called a sigmoidoscope to view the rectum and lower colon. First, the doctor examines the rectum with a gloved, lubricated finger. Then, the sigmoidoscope is inserted through the anus into the rectum and lower colon. The procedure may cause a mild sensation of wanting to move the bowels and abdominal pressure. Sometimes the doctor fills the organs with air to get a better view. The air may cause mild cramping.

To perform a colonoscopy, the doctor uses a flexible tube with a light on the end called a colonoscope to view the entire colon. This tube is longer than a sigmoidoscope. The same bowel cleansing used for the barium x-ray is needed to clear the bowel of waste. The patient is lightly sedated before the exam. During the exam, the patient lies on his or her side and the doctor inserts the tube through the anus and rectum into the colon. If an abnormality is seen, the doctor can use the colonoscope to remove a small piece of tissue for examination (biopsy). The patient may feel gassy and bloated after the procedure.

Colorectal Transit Study

This test, reserved for those with chronic constipation, shows how well food moves through the colon. The patient swallows capsules containing small markers, which are visible on x-ray. The movement of the markers through the colon is monitored with abdominal x-rays taken several times 3 to 7 days after the capsule is swallowed. The patient follows a high-fiber diet during the course of this test.

Anorectal Function Tests

These tests diagnose constipation caused by abnormal functioning of the anus or rectum (anorectal function). Anorectal manometry evaluates anal sphincter muscle function. A catheter or air-filled balloon inserted into the anus is slowly pulled back through the sphincter muscle to measure muscle tone and contractions.

Defecography is an x-ray of the anorectal area that evaluates completeness of stool elimination, identifies anorectal abnormalities, and evaluates rectal muscle contractions and relaxation. During the exam, the doctor fills the rectum with a soft paste that is the same consistency as stool. The patient sits on a toilet positioned inside an x-ray machine and then relaxes and squeezes the anus and expels the solution. The doctor studies the x-rays for anorectal problems that occurred while the patient emptied the paste.

How Is Constipation Treated?

Although treatment depends on the cause, severity, and duration, in most cases dietary and lifestyle changes will help relieve symptoms and help prevent constipation.

Diet

A diet with enough fiber (20 to 35 grams each day) helps form soft, bulky stool. A doctor or dietitian can help plan an appropriate diet. High-fiber foods include beans; whole grains and bran cereals; fresh fruits; and vegetables such as asparagus, brussels sprouts, cabbage, and carrots. For people prone to constipation, limiting foods that have little or no fiber such as ice cream, cheese, meat, and processed foods is also important.

Lifestyle Changes

Other changes that can help treat and prevent constipation include drinking enough water and other liquids such as fruit and vegetable juices and clear soup, engaging in daily exercise, and reserving enough time to have a bowel movement. In addition, the urge to have a bowel movement should not be ignored.

Laxatives

Most people who are mildly constipated do not need laxatives. However, for those who have made lifestyle changes and are still constipated, doctors may recommend laxatives or enemas for a limited time. These treatments can help retrain a chronically sluggish bowel. For children, short-term treatment with laxatives, along with retraining to establish regular bowel habits, also helps prevent constipation.

A doctor should determine when a patient needs a laxative and which form is best. Laxatives taken by mouth are available in liquid, tablet, gum, powder, and granule forms. They work in various ways:

- Bulk-forming laxatives generally are considered the safest but can interfere with absorption of some medicines. These laxatives, also known as fiber supplements, are taken with water. They absorb water in the intestine and make the stool softer. Brand names include Metamucil®, Citrucel®, and Serutan®.
- Stimulants cause rhythmic muscle contractions in the intestines. Brand names include Correctol®, Ex-Lax®, Dulcolax®, Purge®, Feen-A-Mint®, and Senokot®. Studies suggest that phenolphthalein, an ingredient in some stimulant laxatives, might increase a person's risk for cancer. The Food and Drug Administration (FDA) has proposed a ban on all over-the-counter products containing phenolphthalein. Most laxative makers have replaced or plan to replace phenolphthalein with a safer ingredient.
- Stool softeners provide moisture to the stool and prevent dehydration. These laxatives are often recommended after childbirth or surgery. Products include Colace,® Dialose®, and Surfak®.
- Lubricants grease the stool enabling it to move through the intestine more easily. Mineral oil is the most common lubricant.
- Saline laxatives act like a sponge to draw water into the colon for easier passage of stool. Laxatives in this group include Milk of Magnesia®, Citrate of Magnesia®, and Haley's M-O®.

People who are dependent on laxatives need to slowly stop using the medications. A doctor can assist in this process. In most people, this restores the colon's natural ability to contract.

Other Treatment

Treatment may be directed at a specific cause. For example, the doctor may recommend discontinuing medication or performing surgery to correct an anorectal problem such as rectal prolapse.

People with chronic constipation caused by anorectal dysfunction can use biofeedback to retrain the muscles that control release of bowel movements. Biofeedback involves using a sensor to monitor muscle activity that at the same time can be displayed on a computer screen allowing for an accurate assessment of body functions. A health care professional uses this information to help the patient learn how to use these muscles.

Surgical removal of the colon may be an option for people with severe symptoms caused by colonic inertia. However, the benefits of this surgery must be weighed against possible complications, which include abdominal pain and diarrhea.

Can Constipation Be Serious?

Sometimes constipation can lead to complications. These complications include hemorrhoids caused by straining to have a bowel movement or anal fissures (tears in the skin around the anus) caused when hard stool stretches the sphincter muscle. As a result, rectal bleeding may occur that appears as bright red streaks on the surface of the stool. Treatment for hemorrhoids may include warm tub baths, ice packs, and application of a cream to the affected area. Treatment for anal fissure may include stretching the sphincter muscle or surgical removal of tissue or skin in the affected area.

Sometimes straining causes a small amount of intestinal lining to push out from the anal opening. This condition is known as rectal prolapse and may lead to secretion of mucus from the anus. Usually, eliminating the cause of the prolapse such as straining or coughing is the only treatment necessary. Severe or chronic prolapse requires surgery to strengthen and tighten the anal sphincter muscle or to repair the prolapsed lining.

Constipation may also cause hard stool to pack the intestine and rectum so tightly that the normal pushing action of the colon is not enough to expel the stool. This condition, called fecal impaction, occurs most often in children and older adults. An impaction can be softened with mineral oil taken by mouth and an enema. After softening the impaction, the doctor may break up and remove part of the hardened stool by inserting one or two fingers in the anus.

Diet, Stress & Irritable Bowel Syndrome (IBS)

How Do Diet & Stress Affect Irritable Bowel Syndrome (IBS)?

The potential for abnormal function of the colon is always present in people with IBS, but a trigger also must be present to cause symptoms. The most likely culprits seem to be diet and emotional stress. Many people report that their symptoms occur following a meal or when they are under stress. No one is sure why this happens, but scientists have some clues.

Eating causes contractions of the colon. Normally, this response may cause an urge to have a bowel movement within 30 to 60 minutes after a meal. In people with IBS, the urge may come sooner with cramps and diarrhea.

The strength of the response is often related to the number of calories in a meal and especially the amount of fat in a meal. Fat in any form (animal or vegetable) is a strong stimulus of colonic contractions after a meal. Many foods contain fat, especially meats of all kinds, poultry skin, whole milk, cream, cheese, butter, vegetable oil, margarine, shortening, avocados, and whipped toppings.

Stress also stimulates colonic spasm in people with IBS. This process is not completely understood, but scientists point out that the colon is controlled partly by the nervous system. Stress reduction (relaxation) training or counseling and support help relieve IBS symptoms in some people. However, doctors are quick to note that this does not mean IBS is the result of a personality disorder. IBS is at least partly a disorder of colon motility.

How Does A Good Diet Help IBS?

For many people, eating a proper diet lessens IBS symptoms. Before changing your diet, it is a good idea to keep a journal noting which foods seem to cause distress. Discuss your findings with your doctor. You also may want to consult a registered dietitian, who can help you make changes in your diet. For instance, if dairy products cause your symptoms to flare up, you can try eating less of those foods. Yogurt might be tolerated better because it contains organisms that supply lactase, the enzyme needed to digest lactose, the sugar found in milk products. Because dairy products are an important source of calcium and other nutrients that your body needs, be sure to get adequate nutrients in the foods that you substitute.

Dietary fiber may lessen IBS symptoms in many cases. Whole grain breads and cereals, beans, fruits, and vegetables are good sources of fiber. Consult your doctor before using an over-the-counter fiber supplement. High-fiber diets keep the colon mildly distended, which may help to prevent spasms from developing. Some forms of fiber also keep water in the stools, thereby preventing hard stools that are difficult to pass. Doctors usually recommend that you eat just enough fiber so that you have soft, easily passed, and painless bowel movements. High-fiber diets may cause gas and bloating, but within a few weeks, these symptoms often go away as your body adjusts to the diet.

Large meals can cause cramping and diarrhea in people with IBS. Symptoms may be eased if you eat smaller meals more often or just eat smaller portions. This should help, especially if your meals are low in fat and high in carbohydrates such as pasta, rice, whole-grain breads and cereals, fruits, and vegetables.

Traveler's Diarrhea

Traveler's diarrhea is a problem that mainly affects people who travel to developing countries. Diarrhea-causing bacteria live in the water in many developing countries. Visitors often experience diarrhea when they drink tap water, use ice cubes, or eat fruits and vegetables washed in tap water. Less common causes of traveler's diarrhea are jet lag, altitude changes, medicines, or changes in diet and eating pattern.

Symptoms are three or more loose stools in 24 hours. More severe cases will have blood in the stool, vomiting, cramps, fever, or nausea. The diarrhea usually lasts 3 to 4 days. It is not life-threatening except for infants, who may become dehydrated.

A doctor may prescribe medicine to kill the bacteria or to relieve symptoms. The most important part of treatment is to drink lots of fluids to prevent dehydration. Travelers can drink bottled water, fruit juice, or caffeine-free soda (caffeine can worsen diarrhea). If dehydration does occur, the person must drink a special rehydration solution that contains the right mix of sodium, potassium, chloride, sugar, and water.

Lactose intolerance

Lactose intolerance is the inability to digest significant amounts of lactose, the predominant sugar of milk. This inability results from a shortage of the enzyme lactase, which is normally produced by the cells that line the small intestine. Lactase breaks down milk sugar into simpler forms that can then be absorbed into the bloodstream. When there is not enough lactase to digest the amount of lactose consumed, the results, although not usually dangerous, may be very distressing. While not all persons deficient in lactase have symptoms, those who do are considered to be lactose intolerant.

Common symptoms include nausea, cramps, bloating, gas, and diarrhea, which begin about 30 minutes to 2 hours after eating or drinking foods containing lactose. The severity of symptoms varies depending on the amount of lactose each individual can tolerate.

Some causes of lactose intolerance are well known. For instance, certain digestive diseases and injuries to the small intestine can reduce the amount of enzymes produced. In rare cases, children are born without the ability to produce lactase. For most people, though, lactase deficiency is a condition that develops naturally over time. After about the age of 2 years, the body begins to produce less lactase. However, many people may not experience symptoms until they are much older.

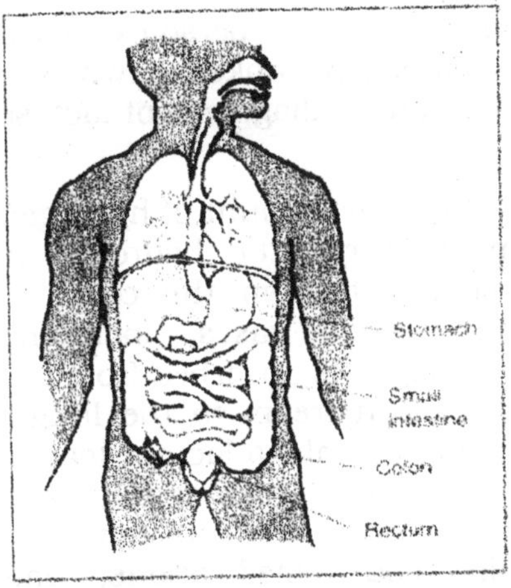

Between 30 and 50 million Americans are lactose intolerant. Certain ethnic and racial populations are more widely affected than others. As many as 75 percent of all African Americans and American Indians and 90 percent of Asian Americans are lactose intolerant. The condition is least common among persons of northern European descent.

Researchers have identified a genetic variation associated with lactose intolerance; this discovery may be useful in developing a diagnostic test to identify people with this condition.

How Is Lactose Intolerance Diagnosed? The most common tests used to measure the absorption of lactose in the digestive system are the lactose tolerance test, the hydrogen breath test, and the stool acidity test. These tests are performed on an outpatient basis at a hospital, clinic, or doctor's office.

The lactose tolerance test begins with the individual fasting (not eating) before the test and then drinking a liquid that contains lactose. Several blood samples are taken over a 2-hour period to measure the person's blood glucose (blood sugar) level, which indicates how well the body is able to digest lactose.

Normally, when lactose reaches the digestive system, the lactase enzyme breaks it down into glucose and galactose. The liver then changes the galactose into glucose, which enters the bloodstream and raises the person's blood glucose level. If lactose is incompletely broken down, the blood glucose level does not rise and a diagnosis of lactose intolerance is confirmed.

The hydrogen breath test measures the amount of hydrogen in a person's breath. Normally, very little hydrogen is detectable. However, undigested lactose in the colon is fermented by bacteria, and various gases, including hydrogen, are produced. The hydrogen is absorbed from the intestines, carried through the bloodstream to the lungs, and exhaled. In the test, the patient drinks a lactose-loaded beverage, and the breath is analyzed at regular intervals. Raised levels of hydrogen in the breath indicate improper digestion of lactose. Certain foods, medications, and cigarettes can affect the accuracy of the test and should be avoided before taking it. This test is available for children and adults.

The lactose tolerance and hydrogen breath tests are not given to infants and very young children who are suspected of having lactose intolerance. A large lactose load may be dangerous for the very young because they are more prone to the dehydration that can result from diarrhea caused by the lactose. If a baby or young child is experiencing symptoms of lactose intolerance, many pediatricians simply recommend changing from cow's milk to soy formula and waiting for symptoms to abate.

If necessary, a stool acidity test, which measures the amount of acid in the stool, may be given to infants and young children. Undigested lactose fermented by bacteria in the colon creates lactic acid and other short-chain fatty acids that can be detected in a stool sample. In addition, glucose may be present in the sample as a result of unabsorbed lactose in the colon.

How Is Lactose Intolerance Treated? Fortunately, lactose intolerance is relatively easy to treat. No treatment can improve the body's ability to produce lactase, but symptoms can be controlled through diet.

Young children with lactase deficiency should not eat any foods containing lactose. Most older children and adults need not avoid lactose completely, but people differ in the amounts and types of foods they can handle. For example, one person may have symptoms after drinking a small glass of milk, while another can drink one glass but not two. Others may be able to manage ice cream and aged cheeses, such as cheddar and Swiss, but not other dairy products. Dietary control of lactose intolerance depends on people learning through trial and error how much lactose they can handle.

For those who react to very small amounts of lactose or have trouble limiting their intake of foods that contain it, lactase enzymes are available without a prescription to help people digest foods that contain lactose. The tablets are taken with the first bite of dairy food. Lactase enzyme is also available as a liquid. Adding a few drops of the enzyme will convert the lactose in milk or cream, making it more digestible for people with lactose intolerance.

Lactose-reduced milk and other products are available at most supermarkets. The milk contains all of the nutrients found in regular milk and remains fresh for about the same length of time, or longer if it is super-pasteurized.

How Is Nutrition Balanced? Milk and other dairy products are a major source of nutrients in the American diet. The most important of these nutrients is calcium. Calcium is essential for the growth and repair of bones throughout life. In the middle and later years, a shortage of calcium may lead to thin, fragile bones that break easily, a condition called osteoporosis. A concern, then, for both children and adults with lactose intolerance, is getting enough calcium in a diet that includes little or no milk.

Age group	Amount of calcium to consume daily, in milligrams (mg)
0-6 months	210 mg
7-12 months	270 mg
1-3 years	500 mg
4-8 years	800 mg
9-18 years	1,300 mg
19-50 years	1,000 mg
51-70+ years	1,200 mg

Also, pregnant and nursing women under 19 need 1,300 mg daily, while pregnant and nursing women over 19 need 1,000 mg.

In planning meals, making sure that each day's diet includes enough calcium is important, even if the diet does not contain dairy products. Many nondairy foods are high in calcium. Green vegetables, such as broccoli and kale, and fish with soft, edible bones, such as salmon and sardines, are excellent sources of calcium. To help in planning a high-calcium and low-lactose diet, the table that follows lists some common foods that are good sources of dietary calcium and shows how much lactose they contain.

Recent research shows that yogurt with active cultures may be a good source of calcium for many people with lactose intolerance, even though it is fairly high in lactose. Evidence shows that the bacterial cultures used to make yogurt produce some of the lactase enzyme required for proper digestion.

Calcium and Lactose in Common Foods

Vegetables	Calcium Content	Lactose Content
Calcium-fortified orange juice, 1 cup	308-344 mg	0
Sardines, with edible bones, 3 oz.	270 mg	0
Salmon, canned, with edible bones, 3 oz.	205 mg	0
Soymilk, fortified, 1 cup	200 mg	0
Broccoli (raw), 1 cup	90 mg	0
Orange, 1 medium	50 mg	0
Pinto beans, ½ cup	40 mg	0
Tuna, canned, 3 oz.	10 mg	0
Lettuce greens, ½ cup	10 mg	0
Dairy Products		
Yogurt, plain, low-fat, 1 cup	415 mg	5 g
Milk, reduced fat, 1 cup	295 mg	11 g
Swiss cheese, 1 oz.	270 mg	1 g
Ice cream, ½ cup	85 mg	6 g
Cottage cheese, ½ cup	75 mg	2-3 g

Clearly, many foods can provide the calcium and other nutrients the body needs, even when intake of milk and dairy products is limited. However, factors other than calcium and lactose content should be kept in mind when planning a diet. Some vegetables that are high in calcium (Swiss chard, spinach, and rhubarb, for instance) are not listed in the chart because the body cannot use the calcium they contain. They also contain substances called oxalates, which stop calcium absorption. Calcium is absorbed and used only when there is enough vitamin D in the body. A balanced diet should provide an adequate supply of vitamin D. Sources of vitamin D include eggs and liver. However, sunlight helps the body naturally absorb or synthesize vitamin D, and with enough exposure to the sun, food sources may not be necessary.

Some people with lactose intolerance may think they are not getting enough calcium and vitamin D in their diet. Consultation with a doctor or dietitian may be helpful in deciding whether any dietary supplements are needed. Taking vitamins or minerals of the wrong kind or in the wrong amounts can be harmful. A dietitian can help in planning meals that will provide the most nutrients with the least chance of causing discomfort.

What Is Hidden Lactose? Although milk and foods made from milk are the only natural sources, lactose is often added to prepared foods. People with very low tolerance for lactose should know about the many food products that may contain even small amounts of lactose, such as

bread and other baked goods
processed breakfast cereals
instant potatoes, soups, and breakfast drinks
margarine
lunch meats (other than kosher)
salad dressings
candies and other snacks
mixes for pancakes, biscuits, and cookies
powdered meal-replacement supplements

Some products labeled nondairy, such as powdered coffee creamer and whipped toppings, may also include ingredients that are derived from milk and therefore contain lactose.

Smart shoppers learn to read food labels with care, looking not only for milk and lactose among the contents, but also for such words as whey, curds, milk by-products, dry milk solids, and nonfat dry milk powder. If any of these are listed on a label, the product contains lactose.

In addition, lactose is used as the base for more than 20 percent of prescription drugs and about 6 percent of over-the-counter medicines. Many types of birth control pills, for example, contain lactose, as do some tablets for stomach acid and gas. However, these products typically affect only people with severe lactose intolerance.

Summary Even though lactose intolerance is widespread, it need not pose a serious threat to good health. People who have trouble digesting lactose can learn which dairy products and other foods they can eat without discomfort and which ones they should avoid. Many will be able to enjoy milk, ice cream, and other such products if they take them in small amounts or eat other food at the same time. Others can use lactase liquid or tablets to help digest the lactose. Even older women at risk for osteoporosis and growing children who must avoid milk and foods made with milk can meet most of their special dietary needs by eating greens, fish, and other calcium-rich foods that are free of lactose. A carefully chosen diet, with calcium supplements if the doctor or dietitian recommends them, is the key to reducing symptoms and protecting future health.